Simple Health Value

Five Overlooked Lifestyle Choices You Can Make Now

DR. ANDREW MYERS

Printed in the United States of America

Simple Health Value: Five Overlooked Lifestyle Choices
You Can Make Now

www.simplehealthvalue.com

Copyright © 2007 Dr. Andrew Myers

Cover design: George Foster, www.fostercovers.com
Interior design: Nick Zelinger, www.nzgraphics.com

ISBN Number 13: 978-0-9790229-0-6
ISBN Number 10: 0-9790229-0-8

Library of Congress Control Number: (Pending)

Warning-Disclaimer

Health Value Publications and Dr Andrew Myers, Inc. has designed this book to provide information in regard to the subject matter covered. It is sold with the understanding that the publisher and author are not liable for the misconception or misuse of information provided. Every effort has been made to make this book as complete and accurate as possible. The purpose of this book is to educate. The author and Health Value Publications shall have neither liability nor responsibility to any person or entity with respect to loss, damage or injury caused or alleged to be caused directly or indirectly by the information contained in this book. The information presented herein is in no way intended as a substitute for medical counseling.

It is recommended that you do not self diagnose. Proper medical care is critical to good health. If you have symptoms suggestive of an illness, please consult a physician—preferably a naturopath, holistic physician or osteopath, chiropractor, or other natural health care specialist. If you are currently taking a prescription medication, you absolutely must consult your doctor before discontinuing it.

First Edition: 2007

Published by Health Value Publications

Published in the United States of America

To Drew and Elke
Mom and Dad
Amy
and
Shannon

for all their love and support

Acknowlegements

It takes many supportive people to give life to a concept and a book like *Simple Health Value*. To each and every person that has been part of the development of this book, I say a humble and heartfelt thank you.

Thank you first, to the readers of this book who believe in the potential to take their own health into their hands and for sharing this message with family, friends and co-workers. I wrote *Simple Health Value* for this purpose.

My deepest thanks to:

My friends and colleagues from Bastyr University, in particular, Dr. Don Brown, Dr. Elias Ilyia, Dr. Michael Murray, Dr. Patricia Elliott and Dr. Jay Little. Thank you for helping me lay a strong professional foundation and for inspiring me to see the art within our medicine.

My friends and professional colleagues, Dr. Rick Tweedt, Dr. Todd Schlapfer, Dr. Joan Haynes, Dr. Werner Hoeger and Dr. Ted Boyer.

My family, especially my sister and biggest supporter, Amy for your constant friendship, hard work and ever present love.

My grandparents, Grandma Ellen, Mom Mom and Pop Pop and Auntie Mardy.

My good friend and business strategist, Maryanna Young, for keeping the momentum of this project going from start to finish. Mahalo! I couldn't have done it without you!

My friends and business partners Dave Brubaker, Dr. Louis Ignarro and the entire NutraGenetics team—Stan, Cavey, Gary, David and Ken. Your friendship and professional support add so much to my life.

For the Leaders Forum and Executive Roundtable members at Washington Group International for your valuable feedback especially Stephen Hanks, Jennifer Large, Stephen Muller, Donna Lewis and Jana Shields.

To George Foster at Foster Covers for the cover design, Steve Smith and Jeanne Gadd at Steve Smith Photography for the photography and Nick Zelinger at NZ Graphics for the Interior Design.

Many thanks to Tim Vandehey, Kim Fletcher, Sharon Dejarlais, Jeanette Fisher, Jennifer Oppel, David and Mary Beth Hollander and Kim Lock for their input and proofreading at various stages of the project.

Table of Contents

Foreword

You were attracted to this book for a reason. Maybe you are someone who is always interested in ways to improve your life and health, making health and fitness a priority. Maybe you are someone who is overwhelmed to the point of confusion by the vast sea of health information and you were attracted to the word 'simple'. Then again, maybe you are an individual who lacks the hope and belief that significant health and life changes are truly within your reach and you are reading this book in need of a new perspective and some encouragement.

Whatever category you fit into, this book is for you. Whether you are on a great path toward living well or seeking where that path begins, you will find simple treasures within this book that are often overlooked in the modern-day search for the latest health fad. The values highlighted in this book tap into the way our lives and health are designed to be maximized, while culture, tradition and an array of unhealthy lifestyles have chipped away at our ability to recognize (and incorporate) some of the most obvious and significant strategies.

Imagine yourself having more energy for your daily activities and responsibilities without having to focus on a strict exercise program. Imagine finding yourself feeling lighter, mentally and physically, without having used the word 'diet'. Then imagine yourself laughing more often, feeling significant, and finding yourself naturally seeking ways to value others and invest in healthy, significant relationships with new passion and energy.

The most exciting element of the information presented in this book is that any individual who makes the decision to begin incorporating some or all of these strategies will begin realizing the naturally—occurring rewards of these new lifestyle and health habits—changes that will inspire, challenge and motivate you to embrace these new habits as life-long patterns with unending benefits.

My hope is that this investment will be one of the most rewarding of your life. Once you are hooked, don't keep the information to yourself—pass it on to those around you and begin enjoying the ripple effect of seeing those you care about discovering some of the best kept secrets of simple health and a great life. Enjoy your new life and live well!

Dr. Louis J. Ignarro
Nobel Laureate in Medicine
Distinguished Professor of Pharmacology,
UCLA School of Medicine
Best-Selling Author of *NO More Heart Disease*

Introduction

As a physician, I am passionate about health and wellness. In my approach to medicine, I seek to address the causes of disease and not just treat the symptoms. I have witnessed the body's inherent power to heal and for all of my scientific training I am still in awe. In my years of educating patients about their health, I always emphasize that health care is really self care.

There are stark realities that must be faced with respect to our health and healthcare system. It is becoming clear that instead of saving us from disease, medicine should be saving us from ourselves. As the incidence of obesity, type II diabetes and degenerative diseases continue to climb, we must ask ourselves, "Are we on the right path?"

I have spent nearly two decades studying and practicing natural medicine. Through my experience I have accumulated a wealth of practical knowledge regarding what it really takes to be healthy and well. What I have discovered is that the simplest aspects of our lifestyle have an immense effect on our health. This discovery is incredibly valuable, but when I look at healthcare as a whole, it is as if no one is focusing on this critical knowledge.

The fact is that most people do not understand the impact that their lifestyle has on their health. And it is this lack of understanding that is costing people their very lives.

Each and every day we make choices that influence our health both in the near and longer term. The simple, often overlooked details—how much water we drink, the kinds of food we eat, whether we exercise regularly—in our lifestyle are critical to the optimal functioning of our bodies and the foundations of our health.

The power to heal is within you. And unlocking that power is as simple as supplying your body with the basic elements of its functioning—water, fresh food, movement, sleep and oxygen. Provide your body the proper foundation for health and you will enjoy two very powerful outcomes: performance and prevention. With a few simple additions to your lifestyle, you will feel energetic and vital—that's the performance part. And as you integrate my *Simple Health Values* into your lifestyle you will optimize your body's function and prevent degenerative diseases like heart disease and cancer—that's the prevention part.

The goal of *Simple Health Value®* is to offer you the simplest, most basic steps to improving your health and preventing disease. There is no magic bullet, no miracle cure, and no systematic approach hidden in this message. The simplest logic drives the information provided in this book and if acted upon you can add incredible quality to your life.

Chapter 1

Being Healthy Doesn't Have To Be Complicated

It Is All About Adding, Not Taking Things Away

Every day, whether you realize it or not, you make decisions that determine how healthy you'll be and how good you'll feel, often for years to come. Some of those decisions are big, like which doctor to see or what insurance policy to purchase. Others you may barely notice, like what to eat for dinner.

Yet make no mistake: Every single one of those daily decisions profoundly impacts your health.

Ironically, the choices that affect your health most are the ones you hardly think about. They are folded into your daily habits and they're easy to overlook. They get lost in the mix of work, family, school, chores, and all your other demands.

It's those seemingly small decisions whether you drink water before your coffee in the morning, whether you walk the dog or choose to take the stairs, whether you eat your cheeseburger with fries or a fresh salad. Each of these choices have the potential to produce lasting improvements in how you look, how you feel and how you live every day.

Shifting your patterns on these daily decisions isn't complicated. My work with patients for the last decade and a half has proven to me that it's simply a matter of seeing how those choices affect your health and of understanding the power of simple changes to make you feel better, work more productively, and even save some money.

Simple Health Value **is about a basic notion: Good health doesn't have to be complicated.**

Doctors Overlook the Simple Things, Too

When Americans become concerned about our health, we generally turn to our doctors. There's nothing wrong with that; most mainstream physicians are skilled, dedicated professionals who have their patients' best interests at heart.

The problem? Conventional doctors are rewarded for diagnosing disease, *not* for preventing it. Their medical training focuses on drugs and surgery. Just like everyone else, they tend to overlook the daily decisions that dramatically influence your body and how it functions.

That's why healthcare in this country often relies on expensive pharmaceuticals with serious side effects, or risky, invasive treatments. Most of the time we wait until something goes wrong with our bodies, then we grab the phone, call a doctor and beg for a pill to fix it.

Working With Conventional Medicine, Not Against It

Let's get one thing straight. I'm not here to bash conventional, or *allopathic*, medicine. It's changed the world and brought us some incredible, life-saving technologies.

The beauty of *Simple Health Value* is that it addresses an area orthodox medicine tends to ignore: A few uncomplicated practices can improve the fundamental performance of your entire body. They can prevent you from getting sick in the first place, or help you heal faster when you do.

No, my philosophy isn't intended to replace your doctor. In fact, it will actually make your doctor and the care he or she provides more effective. At the same time, *Simple Health Value* is a perfect fit if you embrace natural or complementary care, such as vitamins, massage, acupuncture or chiropractic medicine.

If you adopt even a few of the uncomplicated practices you'll discover in this book, you'll build a stronger foundation for good health. So any healthcare provider you see and any treatment you receive will deliver more satisfying results. In the end, you'll take control of your own health and your own healthcare.

**The *Simple Health Value* approach:
Healthcare is really self-care**

It's Virtually Impossible to Fail

You're an intelligent adult. You don't need to be scolded about what foods to give up or why you should leap out of bed at 5 a.m. and run to the gym. So why is it that so many messages related to health are directed at the negative habits in our lives?

Diet or fitness programs that order you to toss out your favorite snacks or make drastic changes in your daily routine are doomed to fail 90 percent of the time. Let's face it, it's tough to make sacrifices. That's why *Simple Health Value* focuses on adding healthy habits to your life, not taking things away. It's a realistic, effortless approach to living with better health and more energy.

Please, don't deprive yourself. All you need to do is add five easy, health-promoting behaviors to your daily routine. The best part? *You're doing some these things right now.* This "simple-addition" approach makes it nearly impossible to fail. Action equals success.If all you do is sip a few more glasses of water or eat an extra apple each day, you'll see real benefits. You'll have more energy, your focus will be sharper, your moods will be more stable, you'll feel less pain and stress. *You will just plain feel better.*

Of course, the more you do, the greater your results. But with *Simple Health Value*, any step you take is a step in the right direction. No matter which values you add to your daily routine, your body will respond in a positive way.

Simple Health Values Defined

Adopt these five easy, inexpensive practices every day and you will improve your health, well-being and quality of life:

1. Drink more water.

2. Eat fresh.

3. Move daily.

4. Sleep and Rest.

5. Breathe.

Now, I can almost hear you saying to yourself, *"That's it?"* I don't blame you. Like I said, most of us overlook these simple steps because they're part of our normal routines. In looking to medicine for miracles, we ignore the miracle of our own body's intelligence and natural ability to function.

But nothing is more important for your body to perform at its peak than these five core elements. Nothing will improve your health faster and more completely than engaging in each of these practices every day.

Most Health Advice Is Complex – Mine Is Simple

When I speak to people just like you about the five daily practices that promote better health, they usually say it sounds too simple. That always makes me smile. Healthcare today is preoccupied with dramatic stories that make the evening news. However, it's actually *because* these five steps are so easy that they're so effective.

Don't be fooled by the simplicity of choices like getting enough rest and eating fresh fruit and vegetables. When your muscles repair themselves during sleep, or when you absorb cancer-fighting nutrients from leafy green vegetables, complex processes are going on that science is just beginning to learn about.

How Long Could You Survive?

Not convinced that the five *Simple Health Values* are the most critical aspects of lifelong good health? Then ask yourself:

- How long can you survive without food?
  About two weeks.
- How long can you survive without water?
  About two days.
- How long can you survive without air?
  About two minutes.

And while movement and sleep aren't critical for simple survival, lack of movement saps your energy and weakens your muscles, while sleep deprivation wrecks your reaction time and reasoning.

The truth is, you need water, fresh food, movement, sleep, and breathing to function well.

The effects of these five daily practices on your health are profound. Due to the fact that you've been eating, sleeping and breathing all your life, you take the delivery system for granted.

No longer. In *Simple Health Value* you'll find out how easy it is to add one or more of these five practices to your daily routine. You need no equipment, no hospital, no doctor, no medication. And if you're already doing some of the things I recommend in this book, congratulations! This is your opportunity to add even more healthy habits to your life.

Most Health Advice Is Expensive – Mine Is Cheap

Healthcare costs are soaring at an astronomical rate. But while the latest prescription drug might run you thousands of dollars each year, working the five *Health Values* into your day can cost you next to nothing.

Imagine your doctor telling you that you could start a healthcare program that never requires a claim form, never asks for a co-pay and never demands a deductible—one that gives you more energy, controls your weight, reduces your risk of disease, and helps you feel better all the way around. You'd jump at it, right?

That's what adopting these five practices every day can do for you. For just the minor cost of grabbing some extra fruit at the farmers market and a couple more bottles of water, you can produce real changes in your health that will dramatically improve your life.

Most Health Advice Turns Your Life Upside Down – Mine Fits Into Your Life

Simple Health Values work because you can blend them into your day almost effortlessly. You're already eating, drinking, sleeping, breathing and moving, right? Now you just need to make small changes in how you do each one.

That's it. No special diets. No workout regimens. No disrupting your routine.

All you'll need are some memory joggers: tricks to remind you to drink a glass of water or walk to the store instead of driving. Once you have those small changes in place, it's easy to take actions that support your body beautifully. As we go along, I'll share some tips that will help you effortlessly include each one of the *Simple Health Values* in your daily routine.

This Is What Your Mother Taught You

You're almost ready to move on and explore the five *Simple Health Values*. Before you do, call your mother if you can. Go ahead. Right now. Tell her you're sorry for not listening to her when you were a kid. She was probably telling you to do all these things from the time you were in kindergarten. And you know what? She was right.

Simple Health Value does make common sense. That's why it feels so familiar. You already know this stuff. In the back of your mind you've probably always realized that drinking more water, sleeping more hours and eating fresh food make you feel better.

Don't be hard on yourself. Like many of us, you forgot. Overcrowded schedules, savvy advertising and the conventional medical mindset drove these ideas into the recesses of your mind.

Here's your opportunity to remember. To remember what it feels like to live comfortably in a body that's functioning at its fullest. To feel great all day long. To enjoy true well-being.

Most people have forgotten how that feels. Your body was designed to feel and function well. Taking action with *Simple Health Value* will allow you to reclaim it. I'll show you by going back to the basics. You may change your beliefs about health—and you'll surely change the way you feel every day.

The Facts:

- ▸ You don't need a prescription.
- ▸ You don't need a doctor.
- ▸ You don't need to spend a lot of money.
- ▸ You don't need to disturb your schedule.
- ▸ You don't even need to understand how the *Simple Health Values* work in your body.
- ▸ You just need to act.
- ▸ You can take control of your health.

Now, let's look in more detail at the power of each *Simple Health Value*. But first, let me tell you a bit more about me and why I'm bringing you this life-changing information.

Ready?

Chapter 2

Personal Passion
to National Mission

Simple Solutions to Seemingly Impossible Problems

S ome time ago a gentleman I'll call Sam came into my natural-healthcare office frantically searching for help. Sam had been through hell. For years he had suffered from debilitating, body-wracking headaches. He finally began taking a prescription drug for relief. Unfortunately, he became addicted to it.

Sam was already enrolled in a drug-rehab program when I met him, and he was desperately trying to kick the habit. But whenever he stopped using the drug, his headaches came roaring back. He felt hopeless, like he was in a no-win situation.

I talked with Sam at great length about his health habits, his diet and his lifestyle, and I completed a comprehensive health profile. What I discovered was that he'd been drinking no water. Sure, he had coffee, soda and such, but virtually zero water.

"Before you start taking one more headache drug," I advised, "try drinking 10 glasses of water each day." He did what I requested and within days his headaches disappeared. It turns out Sam had been suffering from chronic dehydration all along.

Where It All Begins

Sam is one of hundreds of patients I've dealt with who illustrate an empowering idea: You can control your own health by taking a few simple steps.

Just drinking water completely transformed Sam's quality of life. And the simplicity of his solution is what has kept me so passionate about *Simple Health Value* all these years.

True, I'm a naturopathic physician. Yes, I've spent the last 15 years conducting clinical research and educating thousands of individuals. This book is not about that. It's about you, and how what I've discovered woke me up to the overlooked elements of healthcare that put the power of well-being in your own hands.

For me, this journey officially began back in 1988 when I started studying natural medicine at Bastyr University in Seattle. Bastyr is renowned for having the largest naturopathic program in the country, and a rigorous medical school curriculum. One of my tasks while I was a student was to review scientific literature for physicians (like Michael Murray, N.D., who wrote *Encyclopedia of Natural Medicine*) and other luminaries who were responsible for the rebirth of natural healthcare in America. That was long before it became popularized in the media.

For two years I literally read, copied or summarized more than a thousand scientific periodicals dealing with health and wellness. I looked extensively into the scientific side of natural health. And while I do believe in an integrated medical system based on nutrition, herbal medicine and exercise, that's not what this book is about. This book is about concepts that are much simpler than the majority of "health and wellness" books on the market.

I'm here to tell you a story about where health begins. It begins with the basics. And the basics will make you feel better.

We're All In This Together

You and I face the same challenge: keeping our bodies performing at their best while we rush through busy, crazy lives. Everyone struggles with stress. We search for fresh foods to eat while we travel. We try our hardest to get enough sleep and strive to carve out a few precious moments each day just to take a deep breath.

Yes, in many ways we're like millions of other Americans but starting now we have one big distinction. In a few hours when you finish reading this book, you'll know what I know: Going back to the basics can improve your health in ways you never dreamed possible. That's why I'm so driven to share the *Simple Health Values* with you.

This clear-cut little guide is a direct result of my commitment to help your body function at its best using the uncomplicated systems nature has already provided. I feel a reverence—almost a spiritual sense of awe—for how perfectly we're interlinked with the natural world. Our bodies were designed to be well.

We have developed as a *part* of nature, not apart from it. Biochemistry, physiology and anatomy flawlessly support this simple concept. When you look at your health from this point of view, it's incredible what the natural world offers you to boost your performance, promote wellness and prevent disease.

Conventional Medicine Overlooks the Little Things

Once you change your perspective, you'll see little things you hadn't noticed before. While working with patients, I found that the core aspects of health—how we nourish our bodies, how we exercise, and our emotional status—are almost completely overlooked by conventional medicine.

Again, I'm not here to blast mainstream medicine. But does the conventional approach really make us healthier? Sure we're living longer. But are we living better?

Personally, I know the answer to that in my heart. That's why I decided I had to share the facts about the power of simple, natural tools to transform your health. My passion has become my mission. The result? You're reading it right now.

You Hold the Power

If a good friend told you that right now, you have the power to decide

> ▸ If you'll get sick
> ▸ If you'll need to see a doctor
> ▸ How long you'll live
> ▸ How well you'll live

...what would you say? Would you accuse your friend of being crazy? Perhaps. That's our "don't prevent it, just treat it" culture talking. It has conditioned us to believe that only doctors, hospitals and drugs can help, because our health and well being are out of our personal control.

I'm here to tell you it's *not* out of your control as you have been led to believe. *And it never has been.* You have always had the power to decide how healthy you'll be, how good you'll look, and to some extent, how long you'll live. You just need to realize it and take your health destiny back.

I didn't write *Simple Health Value* just to chatter on about the benefits of eating fresh food, drinking more water, and getting enough sleep. I want to open a dialogue about shifting our culture and your personal health. Together, I believe we can start a quiet revolution that will make us all healthier, and ultimately benefit everyone.

Your health is my mission. Let's take a look at the first *Simple Health Value* and how it can help you.

Ready for a drink?

Chapter 3

Drink More Water

Your Most Valuable Liquid Asset

Water is the single most important dietary nutrient you take into your body. It lubricates your joints, aids your digestion, promotes healthy circulation, clears away harmful toxins and regulates your temperature. These benefits are just scratching the surface of what drinking water will do for your body.

The human body consists of 85 percent water. You're practically *made* of water. Listed on the back of packaged food and supplements, you see all kinds of percentages for things like Vitamin C and folic acid. But you don't see anything about water.

Why is that? Water is not a vitamin or a mineral. You can't get it in a pill. Frankly though, it is far more vital to you in terms of your health and physical performance. Increased water intake has an immediate and positive impact on your wellness. Almost every biochemical reaction in almost every cell in your body depends in one way or another on water.

So if you're looking for something simple that can make a huge difference in your health, nothing beats water. It's easy to get. It's calorie-free, cholesterol-free, and fat-free. It's the world's best natural appetite suppressant. And it's inexpensive.

Water is an amazing health-promoting substance. What's astonishing is now much we take it for granted. Water has been pushed out of our diets by beverages like soda, coffee and juice. How did water fall from grace? Well, with the hundreds of millions of dollars spent to bombard us with advertising for soda and other beverages, it is no wonder. So fill up that water bottle, take a long, refreshing sip, and feel the immediate impact.

Why Water When Other Beverages May Taste Better?

Water is the gold standard of hydration. Sure, other fluids can hydrate you, but nothing does it as well as water. Why? Because water is the most basic element in any beverage. Water contains no protein or carbohydrates. Nothing slows its absorption into the body. Orange juice can't lubricate your joint tissues and cartilage. Milk can't help you digest your food or clear away waste products. Coffee can't deliver oxygen and energy to every cell in your body.

As much as your car runs on gas, you run on simple water. Your digestive system is designed to draw it out of everything you eat and drink. So when you swig orange juice or anything else instead of water, you force your body to work even harder to get the water you need.

I'll say it again. No other drink on earth can match water for the hydration you need. That's not to say you should never enjoy a can of soda or cup of coffee. Remember, *Simple Health Value* is about adding, not taking things away. I'm not going to wag my finger at you and tell you never to sip a cappuccino again. I enjoy coffee shops as much as the next person.

Just understand the true benefits of water and make it your drink of choice as often as you can. That's it. That's all you need to do.

How Much Water Do You Need to Look and Feel Your Best?

If most of what you drink during a typical day comes from anything other than water, you're just not drinking enough of it. But let's be real. The question you're probably asking is, "What's the least amount of water I have to drink each day to be hydrated?" I have no problem with that. The easier it is to drink your daily supply, the more likely you are to do it.

Fortunately, there's a straightforward formula to figure out how much water you need.

The *Simple Health Value* Hydration Formula

1. Take your body weight and divide it by 2.
   So if you weigh 190 and divide by 2, you get 95.
2. That's how many ounces of water you need to drink each day. Now take that number and divide by 8 ounces. So 95 ÷ 8 = about 12.
3. You need to drink 12 glasses of water each day to be properly hydrated.

4. If you work out strenuously, you'll need to add 3-4 more glasses of water that day.

You say math wasn't your subject in school? That's fine. Just figure this: If you're a healthy adult of moderate weight, you need to drink 8 to 12 glasses of water a day. You'll drink eight glasses on the low end if you're a smaller person, and twelve glasses on the high end if you have a larger frame.

You may have noticed something interesting about this formula. The heavier the person, the more water required. The larger your body, the more water it takes to flush out toxins and keep all your body systems running smoothly.

I'll Be In the Bathroom All Day!

Sure, 95 ounces sounds like a lot of water. When I tell my patients how much they need, that's generally their first reaction. Their second is usually something like, "I'll be in the bathroom all day!"

Think about it. If you buy a 1.5-liter bottle of water, then empty and refill it three times a day, you'll consume almost 96 ounces of water. You can do that at work, at the gym, walking, even at dinner.

It's not as hard as it sounds to drink the right amount of water. The trick is to make it a natural aspect of your everyday life.

Now, the part about making more trips to the bathroom does have some truth to it. In the beginning, when you're dehydrated your kidneys get used to functioning on less water. So when you drink more of it, your kidneys have to adjust as your body tries to establish a new balance. That means for a period of time, days or weeks at the most, you probably will urinate more often.

Don't worry. As long as you keep drinking the extra water, everything will balance out. Your kidneys will adjust to processing it and you won't need to go to the bathroom as frequently.

Pay Attention to the Three Cs

Not sure if you're drinking enough water now? There's a very simple way you can tell. When you go to the bathroom your urine should follow the Three Cs:

▸ Clear
▸ Colorless
▸ Copious

Clear means your urine isn't cloudy. Colorless means it's the color of water, not

If You Think, You Need to Drink!

Want an edge at work or in class? Make sure you drink enough water.

Many researchers, like those working with Britain's Water for Health Alliance, have discovered that brain function and hydration are linked.

If you're properly hydrated you think more clearly, have better motor coordination, and enjoy a sharper short-term memory than someone who's dehydrated.

Indeed, British scientists have found that just a 2 percent drop in your body's water level is enough to impair short-term recall and motor skills. Test subjects have said they feel "more alert" after drinking water.

So you're probably wise to take a few long, cool gulps before
• A meeting
• A presentation
• An exam
• A date
• A project with a deadline

You'll find your mind clearer, better able to remember details, and primed for peak performance.

yellow. And copious means you urinate frequently throughout the day. And you release a lot of fluid when you do.

If your urine passes the Three Cs test, rest assured. You're drinking enough water. If not? Perhaps you didn't drink enough that day. But more than likely, you need to increase your water intake every day.

Are You Dehydrated? You May Not Even Know It

If you drink too little water and too much soda, coffee or other liquids, you may not know you're dehydrated except by the quality of your urine. The human body is incredibly adaptable. When you don't drink enough water, your body adjusts as well as it can even though you're not giving it the resources to function at its best.

You probably don't even notice the short-term effects of dehydration, so you might not do anything about it. But over the long-term you can't help but be affected. Many doctors agree that a laundry list of health problems afflicting Americans are either caused by or made worse from chronic dehydration.

If you've noticed any of these troubling conditions...

> Difficulty losing weight
> Fatigue
> Headaches or migraines
> Joint or muscle soreness
> Heartburn or acid reflux
> Constipation or gas
> Allergies
> Asthma

...you could be suffering from the effects of chronic dehydration. Fortunately, the cure is easy. Drink more water. It offers a load of benefits besides getting rid of uncomfortable symptoms.

Why More Water Makes You Work Better

Simply put, drinking more water helps your body systems function better. It's an essential nutrient for almost every aspect of your internal operation. Let's take a look at some of the everyday tasks water performs without so much as a thank you.

- ▶ Water pumps up your blood volume. When you're dehydrated you have less blood volume, which makes your heart work harder. That's why dehydration causes high blood pressure and inflammation in the blood vessels. Head to toe, there are a hundred thousand miles of blood vessels in your body. You want to take care of those.
- ▶ Water is vital for processing food, helping your digestive system function more smoothly (and with fewer unpleasant side effects), and helping you extract more calories, vitamins, minerals and other essentials from what you eat and drink.
- ▶ Water regulates your body temperature. Ever go on a hike in hot weather only to find yourself close to passing out from heat exhaustion? That's your body telling you that you've perspired too much without replenishing your water supply. Water keeps you cool and helps you maintain normal body temperature

through perspiration and the water you exhale when you breathe.

- ▸ Water is essential to your blood circulation, which brings healthy nutrients and oxygen to your cells, and removes harmful toxins and other wastes from your tissues.
- ▸ Water helps your lymphatic system, which is a vital part of your immune system, move helpful nutrients, hormones, antibodies and oxygen through your tissues.
- ▸ Water acts as your body's shock absorber. It protects the organs, including your spinal cord, from shock and damage when you walk, run, fall, or get hit on the football field.
- ▸ When you exhale, you don't just exhale air. Water moistens your lungs so you can breathe. You exhale about 1 to 2 pints of moisture each day. Without enough water your lungs would dry out and make breathing impossible.
- ▸ Water lubricates your joints. Cartilage, which pads your joints, contains a great deal of water. When cartilage is well-hydrated, the two bones that meet at the joint glide freely and easily.

That's just a partial list of all the wonders of water. It's a crucial component of the everyday inner workings of every human body. If you want to feel your best, perform your best and live as healthy as possible, start right now by drinking your recommended daily amount of water.

Unless You Have a Hump,
You Need Water Every Day

Unless you're a camel, you don't get to catch up on your water intake. Your body doesn't store much water, and it needs a certain amount each day. If you get it, you're fine for *that* day. But the next day you have to start all over again.

Each day you don't get enough water, your body doesn't function as well. Staying hydrated is a daily task and you'll soon find out it's a pleasurable experience by the way your body feels.

Six More Surprising Facts
You May Not Know About Water

1. **Your body loses as much water when you sleep as when you're awake.** When you snooze, even when you're lying still and not perspiring, the air you exhale is loaded with moisture. If you live in a region of the country with low humidity or dampness (like Idaho, where I live), the air you breathe in may only be at 10-percent humidity, while the air you exhale may be closer to 100-percent humidity. So you actually lose water while you sleep. So it's a really good idea to replace it when you wake up.

2. **Your body needs as much water in cold weather as it does in the heat.** The same physics that apply when you're asleep come into play in the winter months. Cold air is usually drier than warm air, so

you exhale more moisture than you take in. So next time you're taking in the scenery on the mountain slopes, make sure you're also taking in your fair share of crystal-clear water.

3. **Thirst usually lags behind your need for water.** Thirst is a fairly late symptom in the dehydration process: your body usually needs water long before your mouth gets dry. So if you wait until your mouth feels like it wants water before you drink it, you're probably already dehydrated. Do your whole body a favor and head dehydration off at the pass.

4. **Hunger often means thirst.** Frequently, when your body tells you its hungry, it's actually asking for water. Next time you get a craving for food, try drinking a large glass of water instead. You will halt the hunger pangs and at the same time avoid adding extra calories that can lead to unnecessary weight gain.

5. **Water blunts the munchies.** According to a University of Washington study, a glass of water stops midnight hunger impulses for nearly 100% of dieters. That's good news if you like to make simple adjustments in your life that add up to very big benefits.

6. **Water reduces the risk of cancer.** Drinking at least five glasses of water each day reduces the risk of bladder, colon and breast cancers. Now, that's the news of a lifetime.

Make Water Your Main Drink

Almost nothing beneficial in your body happens properly without enough water. So as we begin our journey together, the first *Simple Health Value* should be as clear as a glass of spring water.

Drink More Water

To do this successfully, you just need to change your mindset to drinking water. If you're like most people, water is usually something you drink when soda, coffee or other beverages aren't available, right? Instead, **think of water as a nutrient,** just like food. Because that's exactly what it is.

Improve Your Face Value

Creams and lotions are fine, but the most important precaution you can take to keep your skin looking younger longer is to drink the water you need every day.

Regular water intake:

- Reduces skin dryness
- Keeps skin cooler
- Flushes away toxins
- Helps improve muscle tone that gives skin a firmer appearance
- Flushes fat from the body to minimize the appearance of cellulite
- Keeps nutrients flowing to the skin

To reduce the effects of sun damage and pollution, and to keep your skin looking youthful all your life, nothing is more powerful than getting your fill of clean water.

A nutrient doesn't have to be something with calories. It's a substance your body needs to be healthy. Water more than qualifies. Look at it this way: *Consider drinking water not merely as satisfying thirst, but as an indispensable part of being healthy.*

Think of water as an essential nutrient, more important than any other single vitamin or mineral.

What You Can Do to Get the Right Amount of Water Every Day

Almost every facet of your health and well being will benefit as you drink the amount of water your body needs. It may be the easiest, cheapest, least complicated thing you can do to improve how you feel, how you look, how you think and how you work every day.

Although it's terrific to understand all the wonderful things water can do for your body, the key is getting yourself to drink more. If you haven't been getting enough water for years, chances are you're in the habit of drinking something else.

So how do you change those habits? If water has been an afterthought for ages, how do you suddenly make yourself consume 8, 10 or 12 glasses of the stuff every day without giving up your other favorite drinks?

Replace one 20-ounce bottle of soda per day with 20 ounces of water and save yourself 91,000 calories over the course of a year. 91,000 calories is the equivalent of 26 pounds of fat. Now that's healthy motivation!

Make Your Life Dehydration Proof

There's a simple way to add the right amount of water to your life. Make it impossible to fail. I've recommended this to my patients for years, and it works: Use little tricks and create systems in your daily routine. You'll set yourself up for success by thinking about water differently and you'll find yourself drinking more of it.

Here are some trouble-free ways you can make your life dehydration proof:

Stash water bottles everywhere. Tuck them all over at home and at work. At your desk, in your living room, in the garage, in your bedroom—anywhere you'll see them and think, "Hey, I haven't had my three liters today." You'll trick yourself into remembering that you need to drink more water. A water bottle doesn't take up much space. And you can keep refilling them, so they're cheap.

Wake up, drink two. Every morning as soon as you get out of bed, drink two glasses of water right away. Over the years I've found that people are more likely to drink more water when they start the day with two glasses before getting distracted. It's also an effective way to control your appetite and rev up your metabolism. So if you're trying to lose weight, you should definitely start the day with at least 16 ounces.

Drive under the influence. Keep a bottle of water in your car. What better place to hydrate yourself than at a stoplight or when you're stuck in traffic with nowhere to go?

Carry a bottle everywhere. Buy a brightly colored water bottle to hang from your backpack or briefcase. You see this all the time on college campuses. They're not the kind of bottles you throw out. And because they're bright and eye-catching, you're more likely to remember to grab a gulp or two.

Drink deeply before and during your workout. You don't just need water after a hard session at the gym. Ideally, you should drink two or three glasses an hour or two before you begin. Then down one more before going into your routine, and another half to full glass for every 10-20 minutes your exercise. Do you work out at high intensity or in high temperatures? Be sure to balance that by replacing electrolytes—you can do that with most sports drinks. Remember, mild dehydration can slow your metabolism as much as 3 percent. That not only affects your performance but also your ability to lose weight. And you certainly don't want to leave the gym without the benefits you worked so hard for.

Order water. Every time you go out to a restaurant, drink water with the meal. If you'd like to sip a glass of wine, great, but ask the server to keep that water coming. Over the course of an hour-long meal, especially when you're wrapped up in interesting conversation, you can easily put away four or five glasses of water.

Try a few of these tips and I'll bet you find it easier than you think to drink 8 to 12 glasses of water each day. I promise you this: After you've taken in the amount of water your body needs to get your systems performing at top form for a few weeks, you won't need any more tricks. You will start feeling so much better and water will be an integrated part of your lifestyle.

It really is the simplest, most natural, most invigorating thing you can do for your health, your looks and your life.

Water Wise: Some Final Tips About Water

▸ Don't wait until you're thirsty. By that time you're already dehydrated. This is especially true for children and seniors, so their water intake should be monitored more closely. Drink water on a regular schedule long before your mouth is dry.
▸ Make water your beverage of choice.
▸ When drinking juice, go for the products with the most natural ingredients. Reserve soda as an exception rather than the rule in your daily liquid intake.
▸ Travel is naturally dehydrating. When you're flying in an airplane, drink one cup of water for each hour you're in the air.
▸ When you're exercising outdoors, try using a handy CamelBak® pack or some other personal-hydration system. They're great for carrying water. So it's available on demand.

You can experience the benefits of drinking more water immediately. It is inexpensive and readily available.

Now let's talk about the rejuvenating, delicious properties of fresh food.

Chapter 4

Eat Fresh

Dieting in Reverse

Travel the world and you'll discover that food is celebrated as much more than fuel for the body. People in other cultures have a positive relationship with food. Meals are savored as part of festivals that entice families to drink in the aromas and flavors, and enjoy the tender process of cooking and eating together.

To have a love affair with fresh food is a wonderful way of living. Yet here in America, our fondness for food tends to be radically different. We are so enamored with the convenience of processed food that many of us have forgotten what fresh food tastes like and no longer enjoy the benefits it provides.

Our bodies are designed to derive our nutrition from fresh foods. It's as simple as that. There is much more to the food experience though, and exploring our relationship to the foods we eat is illuminating. Fortunately, you can easily shift your relationship with food. With just a few simple additions here and there, you can zing with the energy and well-being that comes from adding fresh fruit and vegetables to your daily routine.

Don't worry, I'm not telling you to break up with the foods you eat now. Remember, we're talking about adding, not sacrificing. What I *am* suggesting is that you indulge in your own love affair with fresh food. Enjoy the time it takes to prepare it, cook it and consume it. Trust me, when you learn to love fresh food, your food will love you back.

How Do You Know You're Eating Enough Fresh Food?

Even as recently as the 1950s, we got our food something like this: Farmer Joe pulled his produce out of the earth or off his trees. He drove it into town in his battered pickup truck where he dropped it off at the local farmers market or co-op. That's where you bought whatever he grew, whether carrots or cauliflower. Then you hauled the veggies home where you cooked and ate them within a couple of days. Why? Because you had to; there were no chemical preservatives keeping them fresh.

Even if you had lived in a big, sprawling city, the story wouldn't have changed much. You would have gotten your food from your butcher, your baker and your neighborhood markets. Almost everything you ate would have been local, natural and fresh.

Fortunately, folks in many communities today are returning to that nurturing, back-to-basics idea of food. We're all talking about the same thing here: eating fresh, delicious, vibrant food that gives of its natural energy.

Five to Nine Servings a Day

Federal nutritional guidelines suggest you eat at least five to nine servings of fresh fruit and vegetables every day to stay healthy and prevent cancer and other diseases. That's great advice. You'll give yourself a huge boost in vitamins, minerals, fiber, enzymes and other nutrients you need to thrive. And don't forget, raw nuts and whole grains like brown rice are also vitamin-packed fresh foods.

So if you're eating fresh fruit and vegetables at least five times a day, fantastic. You might try eating even more. Some research shows that ten servings of fresh veggies and fruit a day can directly lower your blood pressure and greatly impact your ability to fight disease.

But if the vegetable crisper in your refrigerator is rusted shut from lack of use, take heart. Deriving the benefits of fresh food may be even easier than you think.

Fresh Food Has Vitality You Can Feel

Imagine strolling into your garden in the twilight before dinner and tugging a bunch of sweet, orange carrots from the ground. You carry them into your kitchen, rinse them off, slice them up and toss them in your salad. Then you serve everything with a splash of fresh virgin olive oil and balsamic vinegar.

Consider this: You're eating food that was alive 30 minutes ago. As you do, those carrots pass their life-giving vitality directly into your body. The less your food is refined, the more nutrients it shares with you.

Now contrast that with the frozen carrots that may be in your freezer right now. They were probably grown in California or some other warm climate where they were yanked from the ground, loaded onto a truck and buried under a thousand pounds of other vegetables. Then they were hauled off in the heat to a processing plant where they were peeled, diced into tiny cubes, and rinsed with chlorine and other chemicals to eliminate contamination.

After that they were boiled and stuck on a frozen platform that was trucked out to grocery stores across the country. Then they sat in a freezer for a month or two before you brought them home and plopped them into yours. Once again they chilled out for a few weeks or months before you pulled them out, ripped open the bag, poured the carrots into boiling water and served them to your family.

Of course, a food scientist would argue, "But we test those frozen foods. They have all the vitamins and minerals and fiber that your fresh food has." I'm not arguing that point. I'm talking about a more subtle distinction regarding the vitality that fresh, living food delivers to your body. That's the real difference here.

That's why you feel so much more vital when you eat fresh food. Your body gets refreshed at a different level than when you consume processed food. The body converts food into energy. The less refined the food, the more energy it provides. Your body also doesn't have to work as hard to get the nutrients it needs.

After you eat, do you feel awake or drained? Energetic or

sluggish? Your answer will tell you a lot about whether you're eating enough fresh food, because fresh food makes you feel alive. You don't get that bloated, tired feeling that comes from devouring a bunch of empty food items.

Your Body Never Lies

Forget the food label. There's an even easier way to tell if you're getting enough fresh food. Ask yourself, "How do I feel?" It's true what they say: You are what you eat. And you'd be surprised how smart your cells are when it comes to recognizing what's good for you.

If your diet is high in processed food and low in

If You Can't Pronounce It, Should You Really Eat It?

Care for a nice bowl of butylated hydroxyanisol? Or maybe some sodium erythorbate?

You have to applaud the American food industry. In just a few decades it's managed to engineer compounds our bodies have never been exposed to and have no idea how to use.

When I work with patients to eat more fresh food, I ask them to do something simple: Read the label on a packaged food product. Just go to the supermarket, grab a box off the shelf and read it.

You'll see something like this:

Tartrazine, Carmoisine, Sodium Benzoate, Diglycerides, Sodium Acid Pyrophosphate, Polysorbate 60

If the list of ingredients is filled with things you've never heard of, how natural and healthy can they be?

fresh fare, you might well experience conditions like these:

- Constipation
- Diarrhea
- Bloating
- Heartburn
- Gas
- Regular illness
- Fatigue
- Weight gain
- Bad teeth
- Low energy

Anything on this list feel familiar to you? Then take a good look at your nutritional habits. Simply adding more fresh fruit and vegetables to your meals can quickly reverse even the most irritating health woes.

You Were Designed to Draw Your Nutrition From Fresh Food

Your body was born to run on fresh fuel. Live, whole foods are exactly as we find them in nature. These living foods give you so much more than basic nourishment.

When you chew and consume a piece of raw broccoli, your digestive system extracts dozens of different components and distributes them throughout your body. It's an ingeniously designed, life-giving process that's only possible with fresh food.

There's also much more to fresh food than wholesome vitamins and minerals. For starters, eating fresh veggies gives you:

- Fiber to cleanse your body of toxins
- Phytonutrients: health-protecting plant compounds
- Enzymes to fuel vital chemical reactions
- Essential fatty acids to help combat a host of diseases

We're Just Discovering the Power of Fresh

Science is just beginning to grasp the wonder of food that's consumed in its natural state. We know food is made up of many things: micronutrients such as vitamins and minerals, and macronutrients like protein and carbohydrates. It's also a fine blend of compounds that work together to help our bodies use every bit of food more completely and effectively.

The statistics on the popular fresh foods website, www.5to10aday.com reports that fifteen of the world's leading researchers in diet and cancer recently reviewed more than 4,500 studies. The result: vegetables and fruit came out on top as the foods most likely to help reduce the risk of cancer.

Fresh Food Makes You Feel Full

When you eat food like brown rice, vegetables or whole grains, you get a load of fiber and water. Fiber helps to improve digestive and liver functions, as well as reducing cholesterol. And together, fiber and water makes you feel full faster.

How does a 60-calorie apple stabilize your blood sugar more effectively than a 250-calorie candy bar? One word: fiber. It forces your body to use calories more slowly and completely.

Once again, here are some of the best reasons to eat fresh food:

- ▸ You get more energy from fewer calories.
- ▸ Fiber and water make you feel full after eating less.
- ▸ Eating less helps you control your weight easier.
- ▸ Your body is designed to process fresh food more efficiently.

So with fresh food you eat less, you feel full and you feel better. Add a few apples slices or baby carrots during the day or try new types of vegetables with dinner a few nights a week. Eating well is simply a satisfying experience that can become a lifetime habit.

How To Get Enough Fresh Food Every Day

Eating fresh food doesn't mean you have to cut anything out of your diet. Just find a few small ways to add whole foods into your life. Are bananas the only fruit you can stand? No problem! Just eating one or two more a day will help you feel better.

There are countless tips that will help you eat fresh every day. For the question I hear most often, "What should I eat?" here is a simple strategy:

Eat the rainbow

That means fruits and vegetables of all colors: green, orange, purple, gold, whatever catches your fancy. Each color represents different nutritional contents. So when you eat the rainbow, you treat your hungry body to a full spectrum of vitamins, minerals and other compounds that make it so vibrant and energetic.

Do you do most of your shopping at a supermarket? Here's another easy tip to make sure you bring home the healthiest food:

Shop the perimeter

In a grocery store, the freshest foods are always around the outer edge: produce, dairy, seafood, the butcher and so on. Do most of your shopping there. Unless you need diapers or toilet paper, stay out of the middle aisles. All that stuff in the middle may or may not be good for your health.

While you're at it, spend a little time browsing through the produce section. Take in the textures and aromas of some of the more unusual fruits and vegetables. Ask your grocer or sales clerk about them. Bring a few new nibbles home and try them on for size. You might make a delicious discovery.

Slip More Fresh Food Into Your Life

Just like with water, if you're not used to eating fresh food every day, it's important to adopt some failure-proof tricks that will help make it easier for you.

Start small and snack. Carve out little spaces in your day where fresh foods can fit in nicely. For your morning snack, try a bag of bright-orange baby carrots. Apples are perfect, too. Start taking bananas, raisins, raw nuts or other simple foods to work. Then snack two or three times a day.

Work fresh food into meals. Perk up your regular dishes with a serving of fresh fruits or vegetables. It's not hard to prepare fresh broccoli to complement your chicken and brown rice. Or when you scramble eggs in the morning, grate in a carrot while they're cooking. Voila! You've just added a serving of vegetables to your day.

Add fruit to dessert or breakfast. As you scoop up a bowl of ice cream at night or dig into cereal in the morning, add blueberries. They're rich in antioxidants and have been shown to prevent blindness. Try strawberries, bananas or other berries for variety.

Shop not just for *what* you want to eat but *how* you want to eat. Buy healthy foods and snacks that are easy to grab on the go.

Put fresh food where you can see it. One of the most effective ways to eat fresh is to put the food where you can snatch it. Place a lovely dish of apples on the coffee table, or tuck a bag of raw nuts in your car. If you can see them, you're more likely to choose the good stuff when you've got the munchies.

Prepare and store salads. If you don't have time to chop, dice and toss, simply prepare a large bowl of mixed greens, tomatoes, peppers, carrots, dried cranberries, whatever you like. Then store it in plastic bags or containers. That way, eating a tasty salad is as simple as open, pour and dress.

Today, do something good for yourself. Treat yourself to vital, vibrant fresh foods. You'll feel better and you'll probably enjoy food even more.

If you'd prefer to push on, let's take a closer look at the next *Simple Health Value:* Move Daily.

Chapter 5

Move Daily

The Power Of Taking The Stairs

For some people, "exercise" has become a negative word. It conjures up images of fancy shoes, back-breaking moves and gyms only beautiful people join. As a doctor, I have to admit, I am a big fan of exercise. But exercise has an even more important ancestor that we've forgotten, and it's called "movement."

A hundred years ago there weren't gyms as we know them today. People didn't go shopping for sports gear. Instead, out of necessity, daily life revolved around activity and movement. In some communities, games and sports were part of the social structure. Individuals worked by hand and traveled mainly on foot or horseback. They grew their own vegetables, cut their own firewood, and often built their own homes. They moved all day, every day.

Today, we've lost the benefit of natural movement with the help of all kinds of machines working for us—everything from escalators and elevators to moving sidewalks at the airport. We drive to the grocery store, light gas fireplaces, and move into pre-built homes. When was the last time you walked to the grocery store? With each passing day it seems like there are more reasons not to move.

But, your body is built to move. Every single function, from the activity of your cells to the beating of your heart to the coursing of blood through your veins, is driven by movement. The systems that govern how well your body operates only work best when you're in motion. Body size, strength, flexibility, and energy are all improved by daily movement.

Shake Things Up a Bit

When I talk about movement, I mean moving as a natural part of daily life. Whether it's walking, dancing, gardening, climbing stairs, or running a marathon. Does a specific mental image come to mind when you think of movement?

Exercise, conversely, has become more of a marketed objective. If you work out a few times a week, at a gym or by running, cycling or some other strenuous activity, bravo! You probably already see major benefits. But for most people, exercise takes something as basic and enjoyable as movement and makes it complex. It turns it into something you have to plan for, schedule into your day, and then feel obligated to do.

Natural movement is healthy. It just flows. Imagine a bubbling stream of water that's clear, sparkling and vibrant. *It's alive.* But if the water's not moving, it gets cloudy and stagnant. Movement affects your body the same way. That's why moving yours every day, no matter how you do it, will dramatically enhance your health.

Change Your Attitude, Not Your Shoes

In this chapter, I'm going to show you how easy it is to work healthy movement into your everyday life, so you get all the benefits without having to drastically alter your daily routine.

Remember, the *Simple Health Value* approach is about adding to your life, not disrupting or taking things away. I'm not going to lecture you about joining a gym and working out 90 minutes a day. You don't even have to change your shoes. Just change your attitude toward movement. It really is that simple.

How Do You Know If You're Moving Enough Every Day?

You'll know you're moving enough every day when it's a regular part of your routine. Do you walk your dog every evening? Do you amble to the grocery store to pick up ingredients for dinner? Do you routinely park a few blocks from work so you can enjoy a 15-minute stroll?

If you engage in a daily activity that gets your heart pumping, gets you breathing deeply, and extends and stretches your muscles, then movement is already a natural part of how you live. You're on the right track.

But if you get short of breath walking up a flight of stairs or meandering up a short hill, you're just not moving enough. Your body is telling you it isn't responding well to the movement—therefore you need to work more of it into your daily routine.

How Much Movement Is Enough?

There's no perfect measurement to tell you how much you should move your body each day. It's different for everyone. Fortunately, your body will send you some positive signs when you're moving enough to function at your best:

▸ You'll have a high, consistent level of energy throughout the day.
▸ You'll have a healthy appetite but you won't have a problem controlling your weight.
▸ Your joints and muscles will be flexible, and you won't suffer pulls and strains easily.
▸ You'll handle stress better.
▸ Your mood will be stable and generally upbeat.

If you've been walking, gardening or cycling every day for the last few years, you should feel all these things. Even if you've only worked movement into your routine in the last few months, you'll probably still notice an array of physical and psychological improvements. Keep going and you'll see even more benefits.

If you can't relate to the positive indicators on this list, you have an opportunity to make movement a part of your lifestyle. When you do, you'll be amazed at the rewards.

It's Just a Matter of Time

Adding hearty movement to your day may make some of your activities take a bit more time. Walking to the grocery store instead of driving may take thirty minutes instead of ten. If finding time in your day is your biggest obstacle, consider two things:

1. If your life is so hectic that taking five minutes to climb the stairs instead of riding the elevator is out of the question, you probably need to slow down anyway.
2. Building movement into your life isn't an all-or-nothing proposition. Start small and add what you can when you can, then build up from there. Remember, every journey worth taking always begins with one small step.

It's worth carving a few extra minutes out of your day to improve your health, don't you think?

Why You Should Move Every Day

Your body has evolved to function at its best when you're in motion. Your cells and systems *crave* movement. Like drinking clean water and eating fresh food bursting with flavor and color, movement impacts every aspect of your well-being.

It also directly affects your moods. You've heard of the "runner's high" that comes from long-distance running? You don't have to run a marathon to experience exercise-induced euphoria. You can get that same pleasurable release by taking a long, brisk walk through your neighborhood, or spending the day painting your house that soothing shade of cream that you like.

Moving your body relaxes you and brings on a satisfying sense of fatigue such as the "good tired" you feel when you know you've gotten a healthy workout. There are studies to prove it. Researchers at the University of Texas at Austin found that depressed people who walked on a treadmill for 30 minutes reported feeling more vigorous and had a greater sense of psychological well-being for up to an hour after the workout.

Studies done by the Center for Disease Control (CDC) show people who enjoy participating in *moderate-intensity* or *vigorous-intensity* physical activity on a regular basis benefit by lowering their risk of developing coronary heart disease, stroke, Type II diabetes, high blood pressure, and colon cancer by 30 to 50 percent. Those are pretty serious reasons to add movement into your way of life. Additional studies by the CDC show that no one is too old to enjoy the benefits of regular physical activity. Evidence indicates that muscle-strengthening exercises can reduce the risk of falling and fracturing bones and can improve the ability to live independently in older adults.

The Benefits of Movement Add Up

Are you still reluctant to move for an extended period of time? Here's a newsflash you'll love. In research studies, the benefits of movement actually accumulate within each day. That means exercising for just 10 minutes throughout the day *gives you the same healthy effects as a good half hour of movement.* That's the beautiful logic of your body.

So unlike the benefits of water or sleep, you can actually *bank* the benefits of movement. Your body deposits the pay-off of any exercise into your daily account, even if you did nothing more than climb a flight of stairs for three minutes. Add a few minutes of healthy movement here and there until you reach 30 in the same day, and you enjoy the same payoff as if you took a vigorous 30-minute walk!

That's why it's so easy to work a satisfying, health-enhancing level of movement into your life: You can do it throughout your day, a little at a time.

The Rewards of Moving Every Day

Just as with any of the *Simple Health Values*, it takes time for movement to show its effects. After all, you don't run for a week and then expect to win a 10K race, right?

Daily movement is an easy, gradual way of blending bene-fits into your life naturally. Stick with it and you'll start noticing a vast range of improvements in how you feel and, eventually, how you look.

Here's another aspect that's so simple, we often overlook it: Movement is freedom. If you can't walk more than a hundred yards without losing your breath, you're limited. If you can hike six miles without batting an eyelid, you don't need your car or even a bus. You have greater freedom to go where you please. And isn't freedom what feeling truly healthy is all about?

Avoid the Diseases That Kill

Do you need more reasons to add a nice long walk to your day? How about this: If you move daily, you're less likely to develop the catastrophic diseases that kill. Most of the illnesses that disable or kill Americans every year—heart disease, cancer, stroke, and diabetes—are lifestyle related.

Research demonstrates that when healthy, life-giving movement is a fundamental part of your daily routine, you're much less likely to become overweight, suffer from high blood pressure, or develop diabetes or cancer. Staying active is good for longevity. That's a fact. You won't live forever, but you stand a far better chance of living longer, healthier, and much happier, with a whole lot more energy to boot.

Send Your Heart on Vacation

We often think about exercise in terms of increasing the heart rate. But when you're in shape, your resting heart rate (the rate your heart beats when you're not exercising) actually drops. And that can help you live longer.

If you have the average pulse of 70 beats per minute, your heart is beating more than 100,000 times per day. Lowering your resting heart rate from 70 to 65 can reduce that by some 7,000 beats per day or 2,555,000 beats per year.

By improving your fitness you also rest your heart, so it works less over the course of your life. And less work for your tireless heart muscle means it should last longer and you should live longer!

So essentially, when you move every day and increase your level of fitness, when you're not exercising, your heart's on vacation. We all know that vacations can work wonders. This one's free, and the benefits are endless.

More Movement Is Walking Right Into Your Life

Any talk of adding more movement to your life has to begin with walking, the original form of transportation. It's been with us as long as humans have been able to stand upright. Walking also remains the easiest and most effective form of movement to build into your day.

Walking involves nearly every system in your body. And it's not very strenuous. Unlike running, you can walk for hours. Any walk, from gently strolling around the yard to hiking up a hill, delivers powerful benefits to your body. It's something you can do anytime, anywhere. You don't even need to break a sweat to improve your health.

So if you're ready to mix more movement into your daily rounds, start walking wherever you can. Do you have a dog? Walk him for a mile instead of just around the block. Stroll to the store instead of driving. Walk to the dry cleaner's, to a friend's house, to the park. Amble to the train station or just a farther parking lot.

If driving everywhere is a habit, attach a note to your car keys that asks, "Can I walk there?" This little reminder is a great way to get yourself walking as much as you can.

When you're ready to graduate to more benefits, try walking up hills, or on sand or soft gravel. Both approaches will help you increase your workload and burn even more calories.

Other Satisfying Ways to Move

If you'd like to add more strenuous movement, you have plenty of options. I happen to think walking, cycling, running, as well as yoga, pilates and tai chi are wonderful. They're natural and relaxing yet they work your entire body, so you can enjoy a deceptively good workout in just 30 to 45 minutes. They also help you focus and calm the nerves. Yoga in particular promotes deep breathing and stretching that brings additional benefits to your muscles, joints and other systems.

Here are some more tips to get you moving every day:

Take up gardening. Pull weeds, plant seedlings and till the soil. You'll get a great workout you'll barely notice. If you have a yard, start mowing, pruning and edging two or three times a week. You'll soak up some sun and get some natural, healthy exercise. Try growing some fruit or vegetables which also enables you to get more fresh food.

Go dancing. Talk about making exercise fun! Swing, salsa or your favorite type of dancing once a week is a tremendous workout. Just like gardening, it doesn't feel like exercise at all.

Take the stairs. Instead of riding the elevator or escalator at work or at the mall, start taking the stairs every time. Your body gets a better workout and burns more calories walking up an incline. Using the stairs at work four or five times a day may be all the movement you need.

Park farther away. Rather than circling the parking lot looking for that elusive perfect space, park at the far end and walk. Trying to park close is time-consuming and stressful anyway, especially at the mall during weekends or holidays. At work, at a ballgame—no matter where you are—park and walk instead. You'll get a good workout and reach your destination while the parking sharks are still circling the lot.

Clean the house. Do you outsource your housecleaning to someone else? Start doing it yourself again. A few hours kneeling, reaching, wiping, and moving furniture gives you a terrific workout. You'll improve your home while increasing your movement opportunities.

Hit the floor in the morning. Remember when I said you should drink two glasses of water as soon as you get up in the morning? Try the same thing with exercise. Before drinking your water, get out of bed and do 20 crunches and 20 pushups. You'll work in some healthy movement before getting distracted by the business of the day.

Play with your pet. Give yourself and your loyal pal a daily workout with some energetic playtime. Toss a ball, throw a Frisbee, wrestle, crawl after each other, play tug-of-war—it gets your heart going, improves your mood and delights your pet as well.

It's a Stretch...

Stretching is a misunderstood form of movement. It may not lift your metabolism like walking or climbing, but it's vital to a healthy body.

Essentially, the more flexible you are, the healthier you are. Stretching lengthens muscle fibers, improves joint flexibility, and actually makes muscles respond better to exercise. So stretching can reduce musculoskeletal problems and prevent injury during sports or daily activities.

Here are some tips for stretching your daily routine to include more movement:

- Always stretch when you're warm. If you want to stretch in the morning, take a five-minute walk to get your muscles limber.

- Resist the urge to push yourself to stretch further. It's easy to get injured being overzealous.

- Stretch smoothly. To avoid muscle tears, resist bouncing.
(continued next page)

The Goal Is to Move Forward

Incorporating movement into your day is only step one of the process. Step two is to steadily add more strenuous movement to your life as you become increasingly fit. Properly done, exercise brings positive stress to the body. It compels you to strive, to push further, to do more. When you feel fit you'll want to test your limits. Go for it!

Remember, "No pain, no gain" is a myth, so beware of doing too much. Pain may be telling you you're injured. That's why it's vital to understand the subtle differences between the soreness that comes from good, solid exertion, and the pain that tells your body it's hurt. Do as much as you feel comfortable doing. Then as your level of comfort rises, add more movement. Find something that works for you and you'll see results.

Even if you are wanting to take a rest right now, let's take a closer look at the next *Simple Health Value:* Sleep and Rest.

It's a Stretch... (continued)

- Breathe and relax. It's natural to catch yourself holding your breath when you stretch. Instead, keep breathing. Exhale as you reach, and inhale when you return to a neutral position.

- Stop if you feel pain.

- Recognize that tightness may be a symptom of another problem. Tight hamstrings, for instance, often signal low-back problems.

Chapter 6

Sleep and Rest

The Automatic Recharge

I f you're an adult, you've almost certainly suffered the consequences of not getting enough sleep. Ever pull an all-nighter cramming for an exam only to sleep through your alarm the next morning? Or perhaps you staggered into the classroom, bleary eyed and barely awake, and blew the test. I've even seen people work very long hours week after week, only to wonder why their bodies break from running on adrenaline and not getting enough good quality sleep.

The fact is, needing sleep is almost seen as a sign of weakness in our society. Sleep deprivation is a badge of honor in professions from medicine to computer programming. Here's the truth: If you exist on stolen naps at your desk, or on gallons of coffee and a prayer, you may be seriously harming your health and taking years off your life.

Sleep and Rest Are Not the Same

In spite of all our efforts to develop drugs that eliminate the need for sleep and rest, they are critical to your body's healthy functioning. To be fully fit, to feel your best, to get the greatest benefits from drinking clean water and eating fresh foods and moving, you have to get enough sleep. And you have to rest your body every day.

Before we really dig into this subject, let's clarify the difference between sleep and rest:

Sleep is the loss of consciousness. You close your eyes, drift off and dream. Your breathing deepens, your body temperature drops, your heart rate slows down and your metabolism quiets. Your brain passes through five distinct stages of activity in the process. When you wake up you should feel refreshed.

Rest is taking 10 minutes out of your day to step off the treadmill of your life and slow down. While sleep is a biological need, rest is a choice. Perhaps you stop and simply allow your body and mind to become tranquil and purposeless. It's the alter ego to activity, the balancing element to a hyperkinetic life.

Sleep and rest are equally important for good health. As children, our bodies literally grew and changed while we slept. As adults we act as if sleep is optional, an inconvenience that interrupts our productivity. Now, I'm not saying you need to be like George on *Seinfeld* and build a bed under your office desk, but tell me, how old were you when you took your last daytime nap?

How Do You Know if You're Getting Enough Sleep and Rest?

It's interesting that most people consider sleep a passive activity. They believe that when you're out, nothing's going on with your body. Actually, the opposite is true; sleep is an active process. Your body manages its systems, its regenerative mechanisms, and its vast array of immune functions. These are just a few of the physical activities it performs while you slumber.

That's why sleep and rest are vitally restorative acts for your body. But how much is really enough? Here's a good guideline: If you get 8 hours of sleep each night, you'll consistently feel and perform better. The truth is, the amount you need varies based on your size and weight, how much physical activity you get and many other factors.

If you're an athlete or physically active, or if you work late nights under a lot of stress, you may need 10 hours. So start with 8, then get as much as you need until you're feeling very refreshed and energized the next day.

Rest is more uniform. If you can set aside two 10-minute periods each day to get up from your desk, stroll to a quiet room or garden bench or even your car, stretch out, breathe and let your mind drift, you'll do very well. If you can steal an afternoon siesta a few days a week, even better. Even two brief periods of rest a day can dramatically improve how you feel and perform at work or school.

Got Clarity?

There's a very simple way to know if you're getting enough sleep. Do you feel rested when you wake up in the morning? If you're getting enough good solid sleep, you'll feel mentally sharp, hyper-aware, full of focus and concentration. Sleep gives you energy.

Although, if you're in bed for 8 hours tossing and turning the whole time, you'll feel it the next day. You'll feel tired and fatigued. Every task will be harder. Research shows that the majority of accidents at 24-hour facilities occur on the graveyard shift. Why? Because workers going against their normal sleep rhythms can't help but be impaired and make poor judgment calls.

When you're rested, your mind is clear and your judgment is better. It's that simple.

Snooze Away the Flu

When you get a good eight hours of sleep a night, you won't get sick as often. Say you catch the bug that's going around the office. Suddenly you feel an incredible drain in your energy. That's due in part to your immune system activating and using up energy. That's why you get that overwhelming desire to rest.

On the other hand, if you stop what you're doing at the first sign of illness and you go home and go to bed, your body kicks into conservation mode, directing the energy you'd normally use for daily activities to your immune system. Nine times out of ten you'll beat the illness that way.

That's what makes sleep one of the best remedies for infection. Even when you do get sick, it keeps it from being more severe.

Sleep: The Antidote to Stress

If you're getting enough sleep, you're probably equipped to let stress roll off your back. When you deprive yourself of sleep, your ability to manage stress is compromised. Why? Because your body has no choice but to keep you awake by releasing chemicals that artificially support your ability to stay pumped up and functioning.

Unfortunately, these are the same systems your body would normally use to respond to everyday pressure, so you're already asking your body to go beyond what it can naturally handle. Your tank is on empty. When tension arises the next day, you have nothing left to deal with it.

How do you respond to daily stress? If you handle it pretty well, then you're probably getting enough sleep. But if you find yourself stressed out often, catching more *zzz's* is going to help.

Why You Should Get More Sleep and Rest

Two hundred years ago there was no electricity. When it became dark, our day was over and we went to bed. If you go camping, you may even revert to that natural pattern of rising with the birds and going to sleep shortly after sundown. That same pattern ties into our circadian rhythm, the mechanism that governs our sleep habits.

Today, electric lights and 24-hour everything artificially

extend our days indefinitely. Therefore, we do too. But where rest is a choice, sleep is a biological mandate. No matter how hard you try, you can't avoid it.

It's like a shift change at the factory. When you go from day to night, different workers come out to perform different jobs for the body. Or think of it like living in a big city. When it gets dark and you go home, the folks who take care of your city come out to do their jobs.

With rest, your body works the same way. When you're awake you interact better with the world: You talk with people, drive around town, taste your food and work to make a

Your Body Shop Is Only Open Nights

At night your body is an active system, performing all the maintenance tasks it can't do while you're awake. Here are some of the changes that take place while you're in dreamland:

- Your body secretes human growth hormone, which rebuilds muscles damaged by exercise so they can heal and grow. Sleep is a major component of successful muscle building.

- Nerve-cell connections strengthen.

- Your pulse and breathing rates slow, allowing your heart and lungs to rest.

- Your digestive tract becomes more active. Food moves through it more rapidly and easily, improving your ability to absorb nutrients.

living. Then when you come home, turn out the lights and doze off, those active functions cease and a whole set of new reflexive functions kick into gear.

Sleep Recharges Your Batteries

To a degree, stress will always be a natural part of your life. One way your body responds to stress is by having your nervous and adrenal systems release biochemicals such as adrenaline and cortisol that bring on symptoms like shallow breathing, increased heart rate and hyperawareness.

That's why daily stress comes at a cost to your body's energy, nervous and adrenal systems. By the end of the day, those systems are drained. But when you sleep, unless you have a nightmare, your adrenal glands recharge. In fact, after midnight the adrenals go into rest mode, recharging the same chemicals that give you the ability to handle stress the next day.

So when people say they're "recharging their batteries" while they sleep, they're right. Sleep and rest are the great body balancers that allow you to recover from the endless, hectic motion of your waking hours.

Sleep Enhances Performance

Sleep and rest are nature's best performance enhancers. In the professional world where you're expected to be at your best all the time, rest is considered a weakness. It's ridiculous but part of the cultural productivity status. Research shows that for professional and Olympic athletes who are trying to move up from one level of performance to the next, the ability to rest and get more sleep so that the body can recover is critical to their success. Without the extra sleep, performance will not improve to the degree needed to qualify for the next level of competition or to break records.

The same is true for you. Next time you're on a deadline at your job and everyone else is working non-stop in a panic, try taking a 15-minute break. Go for a walk, sit and watch the birds, and just breathe. Afterwards I'll bet you get more done in half the time and do it with more efficiency.

Clear the Cobwebs

Brain activity is completely different when we sleep than when we're awake. In sleep we pass through five distinct levels of brain function known as the *sleep cycle*:

Stage 1 is light sleep. While we drift in and out and our muscle activity begins to slow, we can still be awakened easily.

In Stage 2 our eye and muscle movements stop and our brain waves slow, except for abrupt jumps of brain activity called *sleep spindles*.

In Stage 3 our brain activity reduces even more and very slow waves called *delta waves* appear.

In Stage 4 our brain exhibits almost nothing but *delta waves*. This is considered deep sleep and at this stage it's hard to wake up.

Stage 5 is that of rapid eye movement, or *REM sleep*. Here our eyes move behind our eyelids, heart and breathing rates increase, and our limbs often become paralyzed. This is the sleep of the dream state.

The average sleep cycle in adults takes 90 to 110 minutes. If you want to feel vital and energetic and if you want your concentration to be powerful you must consistently get enough sleep to pass through all five stages. This enables you to start each day with a mind and body in tiptop condition.

Sleep Floods Your Body With Oxygen

Think about what you're doing for your body when you breathe during sleep. You're breathing deeply, breath after breath, for perhaps the only extended period during the day. When you sleep, you fill your tissues with life-giving oxygen for hours.

Why does this matter? Watch a football game and you'll likely see guys on the sideline breathing pure oxygen. That's because oxygen enhances their recovery. Between the time they come off the field to the time they return, oxygen is refilling their muscle tissues and recharging their ability to perform.

While sleeping, you oxygenate your tissues over and over. You fill your red blood cells, your bloodstream and your tissues with vital oxygen. In turn, you're also detoxifying your body, exhaling carbon dioxide, and flushing waste out of your liver and digestive tract.

A Few Words About Rest

Rest is misunderstood. How many times have you wished you could take an afternoon nap at work? But you can't, can you? Bosses tend to frown on employees curling up on their desks for a snooze.

Here's what they don't know: Even a brief rest during the day can make you more creative, industrious and efficient. That's why it's so important to find ways to work rest into your day.

One of the challenges here is that rest is optional. Our bodies can't function without sleep, but we can still keep going, although not at full strength without rest. One of the greatest things you can do for your body and mind is to take some downtime during the day.

Want to increase your productivity and concentration? Build a pause into your day. Create a moment of peace and stillness to clear your mind, step away from the endless push forward and refresh yourself.

Rest can take many different shapes:

▸ Taking a power nap
▸ Getting up from your desk and stretching
▸ Taking a short walk
▸ Going outside to sit on a bench and stare at the clouds
▸ Breathing deeply for two minutes
▸ Taking a break to peruse the newspaper

The only thing that matters during this restful state is that you take a pause from all the hectic things you're doing. Stop the forward motion and just be motionless for a few minutes. Rest is a powerful tool for well-being.

Want to Get Fit Faster? Rest!

Exercise and rest are two halves of the same equation. To allow your body to capitalize on your workout, you require rest during and after any type of physical exertion. Take breaks while you exercise. Give yourself 60 seconds between sets during strength training to allow your muscles to recover from the work they just accomplished.

After your routine is over, it's also wise to give your body the rest of the day off. Normal movement like walking is fine, but give yourself a break from more strenuous exercise. Your body needs time to recover and to recharge its energy stores as you eat. Proper rest after exercise helps prevent injuries and promotes greater muscle growth.

What You Can Do to Get More Sleep and Rest Every Day

As you can see, it's so easy to take sleep and rest for granted. Our culture has

There Is Such a Thing as Beauty Sleep

Besides helping you feel better, getting enough sleep actually makes you look better. When you sleep you clear toxins from your body, including your skin. And the increased oxygen you inhale carries more nutrients to your skin cells.

The muscles of your face get a rest, too. And as anyone who's had a tough day can tell you, when you're stressed you can feel it in your face. Where do you think those bags under your eyes come from?

So fluff up the pillow and hit the sack for a better-looking you.

drilled into our heads that sleep is a waste of time, something to get through so we can move on to bigger and better things. But, if you know how to work more sleep and rest into each day, you're going to have the advantage at work, at home and in your health.

One of the most practical ways to do this is by balancing sleep at night with rest during the day. If you need to work extra hard and go into a sleep deficit, taking short rest breaks during the day can offset some of the damage. Rest isn't a substitute for deep sleep, but it helps. Here are some more good ideas:

Use sleep aids with caution. Insomnia is a symptom of a larger problem that pharmacological sleep aids don't address. Drugs can't duplicate natural sleep. They don't improve your health. And they can leave you with a medical hangover. They can even be addictive. I don't recommend them. However, there are some natural sleep aids that can be relaxing. Herbs like peppermint, chamomile and valerian are mild, safe and effective.

Avoid stimulants. If you want to enjoy a deep, sound sleep, don't drink a double espresso late in the evening. And don't exercise an hour before bed. Exercise has a stimulating effect that can keep you wide awake.

Get enough calcium and magnesium. Together, these two crucial minerals create a relaxing effect. Make sure you get enough by taking a supplement or eating calcium-rich foods like collard greens and dairy products. Add magnesium-rich sources like brown rice and leafy green vegetables.

Move or workout early in the day. As long as you don't exercise too close to bedtime, it is a powerful way to burn energy and bring on drowsiness. You will feel energized by the movement and it actually helps you sleep better.

Perhaps the best way to handle all this is to build restful and sleep-promoting patterns right into your life. Go to bed at the same time every night. You can even try setting a "reverse alarm" that reminds you when it's time to hit the sheets instead of waking up in the morning.

It also helps to create a ritual around going to bed. Create a short sequence of activities that you do every night to tell your body and mind it's time to relax and wind down. Your lifestyle choices and habits can have the greatest impact on how rested you feel.

Rest Breaks

Since it isn't always easy to slip away for a catnap during the day, here are some tips for getting the refreshing rest breaks you need:

- Create a signal in your office area that says you're in rest mode and wish to remain undisturbed for 10 minutes.
- Read in a quiet place, perhaps in your company lobby or slip away to a non-working zone in your home.
- Listen to soothing music in your car.
- If your workplace or school has a park or greenway nearby, lay on the grass and gaze up at the sky.

- Walk your building's staircase from top to bottom and back again to your office. This works in a bit of good exercise, too.
- Water the plants in your office. It needs to be done, and it's a good excuse to be quiet and walk.
- Sit at your desk and tune out, or write a card for five minutes.

Depending on your situation and schedule, you may be able to come up with many more clever ways to work rest into your days. Just remember, whatever you can do to help you recharge will also help you be more fully awake to enjoy your life.

Your body will appreciate getting enough sleep and rest, and your return on investment will be increased energy and more efficient function out of every body system.

Now let's move on and talk about the final, most essential *Simple Health Value:* Breathing.

Chapter 7

Breathe Deeply Every Day

Stress Is the Disease, Oxygen Is the Cure

More than any other *Simple Health Value*, breathing is something we take for granted. And why not? We do it 15 to 20 times a minute, all day, every day, for all of our lives. We don't even think about it. It's reflexive and automatic.

In order to get the full health benefits of breathing, you've got to understand the difference between automatic breathing, and conscious breathing, or what I call *optimal* breathing.

An Experiment You Must Try

Let's try an experiment. Take a deep breath and then hold it. Keep reading, but be conscious of what you begin to feel as the seconds tick by.

Are you aware that you're not breathing? Perhaps you feel a bit anxious. You see, it's not normal or natural not to breathe. For now, just keep holding your breath. As more time passes, you may begin to feel a more penetrating sense of anxiety that tells you, "You'd better breathe soon or something bad is going to happen."

You can probably see that oxygen is your body's most critical nutrient. While you could survive two weeks without food and two days without water, you wouldn't survive more than a couple of minutes without oxygen.

Breathing Equals Relaxation

Okay, you've been holding your breath for about 60 seconds by now. You may even feel ready to pass out, so release your breath. Discharge all that carbon dioxide that built up in your bloodstream and sent panic signals to your brain. Take a deep, soothing breath of oxygen.

Suddenly, after all that anxiety you felt, you'll probably feel a wave of relaxation with that first inhale. Then, with every fresh breath you take, you may feel your neck and shoulder muscles unclenching and get a sense of your whole body calming down.

That's the sensation you should get from breathing every day. Deep, powerful inhales and exhales revitalize you as they provide life-giving oxygen to all the tissues in your body.

How Do You Know You're Breathing Deeply?

Simple Health Value breathing is a deep, cleansing activity. On a daily basis, most of us breathe shallowly, using only a small percentage of our lung capacity and getting just part of the oxygen our bodies require. It's kind of like holding your breath all day long.

You see, breathing may be automatic, but that doesn't mean it's unchanging. If you lead a busy, demanding life, you may spend a lot of time breathing shallowly while you're under stress. That kind of breathing can become a habit. Even when you're not under stress, you may still breathe as if you are, unless you take conscious control of the process. That's what I'm recommending to you.

The key idea here is to purposely slow down and think about the fact that you need to breathe to take in more oxygen. It's about remembering that every single time you take a breath, you're conducting a health-giving activity.

More than any other *Simple Health Value*, breathing is about training your mind to think in a different way, then acting on that training. It's about making purposeful, optimal breathing a daily habit.

Exhale Your Stress

What's one sign that you're breathing deeply enough? You don't yawn all the time. Scientists aren't a hundred percent sure why we yawn, but it's widely accepted as your body's way of bringing more air into your lungs and up through your brain. So if you're using all your lung capacity, you don't need to yawn as often.

Even more interesting is the chicken-and-egg situation that comes with stress. When you're under pressure, your breathing becomes shallow and faster. It's not clear whether the stress causes the shallow breathing, or whether you become more anxious because you're not getting enough oxygen.

Either way, the connection is clear: If you generally don't get stressed-out, you're probably breathing deeply and often enough to shed the anxiety. On the flip side, if you constantly have a hard time dealing with stress, you're probably breathing too shallowly and denying your body the nutritious oxygen it needs to handle tough situations.

Feed Your Head

Another way you know you're breathing optimally is that your mental performance is clear and sharp. Your brain needs a tremendous, continuous flow of oxygen to continue running the vast network of systems in your body. When you breathe deeply, you super-oxygenate your brain tissues and give them fuel to work powerfully. Your

Breathing 101

If you suffer from anxiety, you may tend to breathe shallowly from your chest. This can lead to hyperventilation since your body needs to breathe faster to get enough oxygen. So learning to breathe correctly is as important as remembering to breathe deeply.

Take a breath and watch yourself. Are your chest and shoulders moving? If so, you're breathing from your chest. But true deep breathing comes from the diaphragm, which is located in your lower abdomen.

Try this:

- Place one hand below your navel.
- Inhale slowly and deeply through your nose. Imagine that your abdomen is a balloon slowly inflating from the bottom up. Feel the air filling your lower abdomen first.
- Count slowly to three and feel your hand rise.
- If you watch, you should see your belly moving out and down. That's when you know you're breathing for maximum benefit.

cognitive skills are faster, your senses keener and your thinking swifter.

Habitual shallow breathers, on the other hand, have a tougher time getting the thought processes going because their brains are crying out like Oliver Twist: "Please, sir, can I have some more?" If your thinking isn't as agile as you'd like, start taking time out to breathe deeply.

Why You Should Breathe Deeply Every Day

Every cell in your body needs oxygen. The reason we each have a heart and cardiovascular system is to deliver oxygen to our cells, which use it as a catalyst for the chemical reactions that turn food into energy. Oxygen is life.

So while other systems of the body are important, they all depend on oxygen. Eating fresh food, drinking water, getting plenty of sleep and rest, and moving your body every day will only have a beneficial impact on your health if you're breathing. Breath is the foundation of life.

Research done at Baylor University shows that lack of oxygen is a major cause of heart disease, stroke and cancer. Simple deep breathing daily along with moderate activity can reverse the effects of these lifestyle-related diseases. Another important fact to note is that the brain requires more oxygen than any other organ. If it doesn't get enough, the result is mental sluggishness, negative thoughts, depression, and eventually, vision and hearing decline.

Chemistry Gone Wild: Your Body Under Stress

Stress isn't just an excuse for not being able to perform under pressure. Your body's stress response, which evolved to help you survive danger, involves specific processes that can actually damage your body over the long term.

The most notable involves the release of cortisol, a hormone produced in the adrenal glands. When you're in an agitated state, cortisol floods into your bloodstream.

While cortisol has a wide range of effects, when you're under stress it increases your heart rate, elevates your blood pressure, speeds up your breathing, rushes blood to your brain and vital organs, and does everything it can to ready your body for "fight or flight."

It's not hard to see how remaining under stress can damage your body. At the same time, your body has a natural control mechanism for these responses –breathing.

Your Best Defense

What's the best reason to set aside five minutes every day to breathe deeply? Simply put, it's your body's best immediate defense against stress. Even if you're in the middle of a tense situation, you can develop the awareness to know when your breathing is fast and shallow. And you can immediately start taking long, slow, deep breaths and actually fool your body into thinking the stress has passed.

When you take even a single hearty breath, your body gets the signal to quit releasing adrenaline, cortisol and other stress hormones. Your heart rate and blood pressure can even drop in response. That's right. One deep breath can stop the stress response, while multiple deep breaths can reverse its effects.

It's a beautiful self-fulfilling prophecy: If you trick your body into thinking a stressful situation is over even when you're in the middle of it, you become more clear-headed and capable, thus being able to resolve the source of the stress faster, all thanks to a few relaxing breaths.

Chemistry Gone Wild: Your Body Under Stress

Your cardiovascular system responds to oxygen. So taking some long, deep breaths can slow or even turn off your stress response and reduce your heart rate and blood pressure.

That's why deep breathing is such an effective tool to minimize the harmful effects of chronic stress on your body.

Exhaling Stress

Imagine that each day our stress was compressed into a pebble—we'll call it our "pebble of stress." You have two choices as to what you can do with your daily pebble of stress. You can throw that pebble away or you can place it in your backpack. Now you might ask yourself, "What's the big deal about a pebble?" But multiply that pebble by 365 days and it starts to feel like a rock. Multiply that rock by 10 years and it's like hauling a boulder around on your back. Suddenly your backpack bends you to the ground. It's an effort just to stand. Your shoulders ache under the pressure. That's how you feel after your body has endured years of unrelenting stress.

Breathing Peels Away Layers of Pressure

The act of deep breathing is all about reducing the effects of stress. You can use deep breathing therapeutically as a mechanism to enhance your health. Five or ten deep breaths a day can help you drop that pebble so you don't end up with a boulder on your back.

At the heart of deep breathing is the simple act of taking time out to do it, which dovetails nicely with your everyday need for sleep and rest. By taking a few minutes out of each day to sit quietly, breathe deeply and fill your body with oxygen, you'll experience an improvement in your ability to handle stress. And that will translate into real, long-term health and lifestyle benefits.

How to Breathe More Every Day

Breathing is the one *Simple Health Value* that doesn't require another object, like food or time that must be devoted to it alone, like sleeping. You already breathe all the time. Getting the real benefits just means changing how you do it.

My recommendation is as simple as this: First, take a few minutes a day to breathe deeply and second, use simple, optimal breathing whenever you feel stressed. That's when your body most needs it.

Certainly, every breath you take fulfills your body's need for oxygen. But when you feel particularly stressed, use deep breathing as a tool to lower the impact of that stress on your body.

Personally, I consider "stress management" an oxymoron. You often have little control over the pressures that come into your life. But what you can do is equip your body to offset the impact of that stress.

Taking five or ten deep breaths in a row, breathing in through your nose and out through your mouth, actually affects your body biochemically, leading to a relaxing, calming effect that goes beyond a simple break in your day.

Here are some more ideas for getting yourself to breathe actively:

Devote five minutes a day to deep breathing. Block out a few minutes every day, perhaps at work where you may get the most stressed, to breathe deeply. You might need to slip away to a quiet spot and breathe with your eyes closed. Or perhaps you can continue working at your computer, breathing deeply while you do. Either way, you'll feel immediate benefits. Start with five or ten deep breaths in a row, then expand to five minutes a day. If it helps, set a specific time each day as your "breathing break."

Integrate activities that facilitate movement and breathing such as yoga or stretching. Try techniques like visualization or biofeedback along with your breathing.

Breathe deeply during slow- or moderate-paced walking. This enables you to make deep breathing an automatic addition to your lifestyle.

Unfortunately, aside from the five minutes a day I'm asking you to devote to deep breathing, your breathing during the other 1,435 minutes of your day is likely to be reflexive and shallow. So here are a few more valuable tips for breathing deeply throughout the rest of your day:

Create visual cues. Decide on a specific set of visual triggers—things that will remind you to take two or three lung-filling breaths. They can be anything from a specific color to certain road signs, or any man who's wearing glasses. You'll see the cues at least a few times a day, making this is a highly effective trick for remembering to breathe deeply.

Create sound cues. Form a set of sound triggers that work just like visual cues. Make a list of sounds that remind you to breathe when you hear them. You may choose the sound of your alarm clock, a car honking its horn, or your cell phone ringing.

Breathe deeply during other activities. Inhale long and deep while you're doing other things, like taking a shower, sitting in traffic, preparing dinner, or a dozen other moments when you can grab a few good deep breaths.

As you retrain your body to breathe deeply, it will become a reflex. You'll begin to overcome your usual stress response and teach your body to breathe more completely. More importantly, you'll reduce the harsh impact of stress on your long-term health.

Now, let's take a quick look at the many ways each *Simple Health Value* benefits you.

Chapter 8

Simple Health Benefits

How Five Overlooked Daily Practices
Can Give You the Energy to Soar

Congratulations! You've just completed a basic course in the five *Simple Health Values*. You've read about how adding each of these easy-to-follow practices to your daily life can improve how you feel, look and live for years to come.

Now let's get to the heart of the matter: the specific ways each *Simple Health Value* can benefit your body.

The Benefits of Drinking Enough Water

Appetite suppression–When your body tells you it's hungry, what it often craves is water. Drinking one or two glasses of water when you feel hungry can keep you from overeating.

Weight loss–Water helps the body metabolize stored fat and flush it out of the body. If you're not drinking enough water, your body retains fluid to compensate. Drinking more water reestablishes the balance and stimulates the kidneys, so it actually prevents you from retaining water.

Skin protection–Sun dehydrates the skin. If you want to beautify your skin and look younger throughout your life, drink water before, during and after each exposure to the sun.

Heartburn and acid reflux prevention–Drinking enough water can prevent many uncomfortable bouts of acid reflux and heartburn.

Muscle development–When you exercise you produce lactic acid, which makes your muscles feel fatigued. To grow new muscle you've got to flush out that lactic acid. Water does the trick.

Less joint pain–Many physicians now think one of the main causes of arthritis may be decades of chronic dehydration, which allows cartilage to wear faster. Keeping hydrated can reduce joint pain in the short term, and may prevent arthritis in the long run.

Better vaginal lubrication–Drinking water can even improve the sexual experience for women.

Easier pregnancy and nursing–Women who drink more water produce more amniotic fluid, which gives babies a healthier, safer environment in which to grow. It also helps prevent morning sickness, and it helps nursing moms produce more breast milk.

Better prostate health–Water promotes healthy urination. And it can lower the risk of bladder infections and kidney problems, which are often linked to an enlarged prostate.

Relief from asthma symptoms–Histamine is often what sets off an asthmatic reaction. As people with asthma become more dehydrated, their histamine levels rise. The body's defense is to close down the airways. Drinking water regularly helps to prevent this.

The Benefits of Eating Fresh

You don't have to eat up to nine servings of fresh fruit and vegetables every day to see the benefits. Even a few extra fresh food servings deliver serious short-term gifts:

More energy–Eating whole, natural, unrefined foods gives your body the kind of energy it was built to use, as well as fiber, enzymes and other nutrients that help your body make better use of food energy.

Improved digestion–Eating whole vegetables and fruit with the skin on adds fiber to your diet. Fiber can also reduce or eliminate problems with gas, constipation, heartburn and indigestion.

Better immune function–When you're flooding your body with essential vitamins, minerals and key compounds, you'll find you get sick less often. And even when you do get sick, it will generally last for a shorter time.

Even better are the major, long-term benefits of eating fresh. It helps prevent the lifestyle diseases that kill us:

Cancer–Whole fruits, vegetables, grains and legumes help you fight the cellular damage that can lead to cancer. They decrease hormones that are thought to cause breast cancer. Eating vegetables has been shown to decrease the risk of liver cancer. Eating onions lowers the rate of stomach cancer. And eating foods rich in lycopene, found in tomatoes, lowers the risk of prostate cancer.

Heart disease–A diet high in fiber and low in fat has been proven to reduce the risk of cardiovascular disease.

Arthritis–Antioxidants, like the ones you get eating foods such as blueberries and peppers, are thought to slow the breakdown of joint cartilage.

Osteoporosis–Eating calcium-rich foods like spinach and broccoli helps seniors and post-menopausal women avoid the bone loss that leads to osteoporosis.

Blindness–Scientific research has shown that eating fruits, vegetables and whole grains translates into a lower risk of cataracts.

The Benefits of Moving Daily

Higher metabolism–When you move regularly, you increase your metabolism. As a result, your body burns more calories, making it easier to lose weight and keep it off.

Better cardiovascular health–Movement makes your heart work harder, strengthening your heart muscle and bringing more blood and oxygen to your tissues. The result? A healthier, more efficient cardiovascular system.

Lower blood pressure–Regular movement widens your blood vessels, leading to lower blood pressure. The weight loss that daily movement provides also lowers blood pressure.

Improved mood–Exercise is proven to relieve many of the symptoms of depression. If you're feeling down, take a walk. It might be all you need to begin feeling better.

Improved flexibility–Movement improves muscle flexibility, range of motion, and the lubrication of your joints.

Greater endurance–Moving daily gradually boosts the oxygen level in your bloodstream, which is a key element of endurance. Regular movement will give you the endurance to be able to play with your kids, romp with your dog, take a walk at sunset and feel better afterwards.

Reduced menopause symptoms–Research shows that women of menopausal age typically experience fewer symptoms such as hot flashes and night sweats when they're exercising consistently.

The Benefits of Sleep and Rest

There are few aspects of your health that don't benefit from getting more sleep and rest. It's an easy cure-all that's already built into your life. Here are some of the benefits:

Greater vitality–When you're fully rested you're vital and energized, and your senses are more vivid. Vitality means you have a higher level of energy and you can accomplish more in less time.

You feel awake–This seems like an obvious benefit but vital nonetheless. When you're getting enough sleep, there's no veil of fatigue between you and the world. Instead, your consciousness is crisp and your thoughts are clear.

Greater stamina–You have more stamina and strength when you're fully rested. You'll also better enjoy the full benefits of an aerobic or anaerobic workout with a healthy night's sleep.

Reduced rate of injury–Tired muscles pull more easily, tired joints tear ligaments more readily, and a fatigued back is more likely to sustain an injury.

Less pain–When you sleep, you flood the body with oxygen, recharge the adrenal glands, and relax the muscles and joints, all of which help you relieve pain and heal.

Sharper mental performance–Being rested improves your judgment, your reaction time, your concentration, your memory and your analytical skills.

Improved athletic performance–You can only exercise a muscle so much before it breaks down. Sleep repairs torn muscle fibers, eliminates carbon dioxide and lactic acid, and floods muscles with nutrients, making peak athletic performance possible.

Stable blood sugar–Your body expends less energy during sleep, so it's better able to control and regulate the release of blood sugar. That can translate into a more stable metabolism and better weight control.

The Benefits of Optimal Breathing

Breathing deeply provides two types of benefits. The first is the reward of oxygenating your body:

Improved ability to handle stress–Chronic stress contributes to heart disease and high-blood pressure. The chemicals the body releases that respond to stress make harsh demands on the heart, blood vessels and other systems. When the body gets plenty of oxygen through deep breathing, it releases less of these stress-related chemicals. That gives your body a chance to slow down, recharge and relax.

Better performance from every body system–When you saturate your body tissues with oxygen, all your systems, from your muscles to your brain to your digestive tract, function more efficiently.

Faster recovery–If your tissues are oxygenated, you're able to bounce back faster from a day of hard work or recreational activities. The extra oxygen helps speed healing throughout your body.

More satisfying sleep–Better breathing translates to deeper, more undisturbed, more restful sleep, because your body isn't sending out warning signals about a lack of oxygen.

The second is the stress-reduction benefit of regular deep breathing:

Reduced flow of stress hormones–Deep breathing reverses the effects of stress by halting the flow of hormones that constrict blood vessels, increase heart rate, and bring on the "fight or flight" reaction.

Slowed heart rate–A few deep, cleansing breaths will slow your pulse. As more oxygen floods into your lungs, your heart doesn't have to work so hard to supply oxygen to your tissues.

Clearer thinking–Reversing the stress response and giving your brain a fresh flow of oxygen clears your mind of distractions.

Greater concentration and creative ability–If you've ever been on a tight deadline, you know how therapeutic it can be to take a few minutes to step away and take some deep breaths. It resets your mind and restores your focus.

Enhanced ability to deal with future stress–Habitual deep breathing helps you stay more composed, controlled and in command of your emotions, all key to dealing with anxiety-filled situations.

Everything Is Connected

As you've probably noticed, all these simple, effective ways of improving your core body functions are interwoven. Just as every system in your body is interlinked with all the others, each *Simple Health Value* feeds off the other four. Exercise is linked to breathing. Drinking more water helps you digest food better. Sleep helps you absorb the effects of a workout to the fullest.

Most of these practices will improve your digestion, your energy, your mood, and your ability to handle stress. When you practice all five *Simple Health Values*, you'll experience an incredible boost in your body performance, your sense of well-being and your quality of life.

Now let's wrap things up by looking at some dawn-to-dusk schedules for each *Simple Health Value*.

Chapter 9
Putting it All Together

Strategies for Building *Simple Health Value* Into Your Routine

You're near the end of the beginning of your journey, and that says a great deal about you. By reading this far you've already proven you're committed to living a healthier lifestyle. Now we're going to place the final piece into the puzzle.

What's the most difficult part about drinking more water, eating fresh food, moving your body, getting extra sleep and rest as well as breathing more? It isn't knowing *why* you should do these things. It's working them into your busy day in a way that's simple, convenient and pain-free.

It's a message I hear all the time from my patients and members of speaking audiences. When individuals ask me *how* to change years of eating or sleeping habits, I tell them the same thing I've told you: It's about doing what makes it easy and convenient to succeed.

In this chapter, that's what you'll find: Daily schedules to help you work each of the five *Simple Health Values* into your life, from the moment you climb out of bed in the morning to the time you go to sleep every night.

These schedules have been built around the natural increments of time that divide up your day such as breakfast, work breaks and activities that occur every day. You can create your own daily routine, including time to rest and breathe.

If the schedules listed here don't work perfectly for you, come up with your own system to produce even better results. This is a starting place to begin making small changes in your routine that will lead to big improvements in how you feel, how you perform athletically, your concentration, your weight, your sex drive and every other aspect of your life.

Drink More Water

Dawn-to-Bedtime Schedule

TIME	ACTION	GLASSES PER DAY
Wake up	Drink 2-3 glasses	2
Drive to work	Sip from water bottle in your car	1
At work	Sip from water bottle at your desk	3
Drive home	Sip from water bottle in your car	1
Before dinner	Drink 2 glasses	2

TIME	ACTION	GLASSES PER DAY
Dinner	Drink 2 glasses with dinner	2
Bedtime	Drink 1 glass at bedtime	1
Total glasses daily:		**12**
	If you exercise,	add 2-3 glasses of water
Total glasses daily with exercise:		**14-15**

Eat Fresh Food

Dawn-to-Bedtime Schedule

TIME	ACTION	SERVINGS
Breakfast	Add fresh fruit to cereal	1-2
	Grate fresh carrot or other vegetable into scrambled eggs	
Mid-Morning Snack	Bring apples/ carrots/bananas (any fresh food you like) to work as a snack	1
Lunch	Eat at least 1 serving of fresh fruit or vegetables	1-3
	Munch on a mixed salad	

TIME	ACTION	SERVINGS
	Try making a new kind of sandwich with less meat and more vegetables	
Mid-Afternoon Snack	Enjoy fresh, raw nuts Eat more fresh fruit or vegetables that you brought into your workplace	1-2
Dinner	Have at least 2 servings of fresh vegetables: corn, beans, squash, whatever is available	2-4
	Serve a salad	
	Focus less on meat and more on fresh produce	
	Savor berries with yogurt or cream for dessert, or top your favorite ice cream with berries	
Total Servings Daily:		**6-12**

Move Your Body

Dawn-to-Bedtime Schedule

TIME	ACTION
Morning	Take a 20-30 minute walk first thing in the morning. Got a dog? Ask him or her to join you.

TIME	ACTION
	Walk or cycle to work if possible
Work	Park your car farther from work
	Take the stairs instead of the elevator or escalator
Mid-Morning	Take a walk around the block
Lunch	Walk to lunch
Mid-Afternoon	Take a small stretch break
	Walk around the block
Dinner	According to an old Chinese proverb, a person should walk 150 paces before dinner and 1,000 paces after dinner. Walk at least 1,000 paces (about 3/4 of a mile) within 30 minutes of eating dinner.
Exercise	If you can, add a regular workout to this movement schedule: run or go cycling. Of course, always walk wherever and whenever possible.

Sleep and Rest

Ways to Get Better Sleep and More Rest Every Day

ACTION	METHOD
Mid-morning rest	Find an undisturbed place near your workspace and sit quietly for 10 minutes, maybe with your eyes closed. Don't read or engage in conversation. Just let your mind drift.

ACTION	METHOD
Mid-afternoon rest	Do the same you did in the morning: Retreat to a quiet spot where you can disconnect from work stress and any demands on your mind.
	Go to bed at the same time every night. Set an alarm to remind you it's bed time. If you must stay up later, make it on the weekend.
	Establish a pre-bedtime ritual Go through the same motions every night. Put on your pajamas, brush your teeth, lay out your clothes for the next day. A routine gets you into sleep mode.

Breathe

Ways to Breathe Deeply on a Daily Basis

ACTION	METHOD
Mid-morning deep breathing	Set a time every morning to do 5 minutes of deep breathing. Remember, you don't have to close your eyes to do it.

ACTION	METHOD
Mid-afternoon deep breathing	Set a time every afternoon to do 5 minutes of deep breathing.

Using visual cues:
Choose certain things that remind you to do some deep breathing. For example, when you're driving and you see a school bus, take two deep breaths.

Using auditory cues:
You can also use sounds to remind you to breathe. For instance, whenever your phone rings at work, you can train yourself to take one deep breath before answering it and another as you hang up. |
| 5 minutes of deep breathing | You can do this during your morning or afternoon rest breaks. Or you can do it in the shower, or as part of your morning commute. Simply set aside 5 uninterrupted minutes to fill and empty your lungs. |

How a Single Mom Holds Onto Her Values

So how this work in real life? Consider Janice a busy mother of two great children who wants to get a *Simple Health Value* lifestyle while balancing work, family and maintaining a productive professional life.

Janice wakes up to the alarm clock at 7 a.m., climbs out of bed and takes a nice, long stretch. Then she strolls into the kitchen and grabs the clean glass she left by the coffee pot the night before. After taking a few deep, cleansing breaths, she drinks two full glasses of fresh water. Then she sets the coffee pot to brew, puts breakfast out for the kids and heads for the bathroom, where she throws on a t-shirt and jeans.

After getting dressed, Janice returns to the kitchen for another glass of water that she drinks with her multivitamin. Then she slices up a banana and grabs a small handful of fresh blueberries to toss over her cereal.

When she's done with breakfast, she grabs the leash and her dog Buster, and walks down the street with the kids to the bus stop. Once the kids get picked up, she circles the block once more before going home. After taking a nice, hot shower, she sits down for 3 minutes of deep breathing before slipping on her suit, grabbing her briefcase and jumping in the car. As she drives the 20 minutes to work, she continues to sip fresh water from the water bottle she brought with her.

Near the office, Janice pulls into a parking garage about a block from her building. While there's plenty of space in front of her office, she prefers to get in a brisk stroll to combat any stress that may be coming her way. Then, instead of taking the elevator, she walks up the three flights of stairs to her office.

Once at her desk she reviews her e-mails and makes progress on a couple different marketing projects. About 10 a.m. she grabs a handful of almonds and a banana from her tote bag, which she eats at her desk while writing a project update. When the phone rings, she takes a deep breath before answering it. After wrapping up the conversation, she continues working until noon, hydrating herself throughout the morning with water from a water bottle she keeps on her desk.

For lunch, Janice grabs her lunch tote from the fridge and strolls down the street to a park. It's a brisk day and the fresh air feels good. She finds a bench, pulls out a tomato and basil wrap stuffed with fresh veggies and enjoys it with a slice of good cheddar cheese. Then she eats a peach, sits back and relaxes. For the next 10 minutes she just lets her mind drift, not focusing on any one subject. When she's done, she takes a few deep breaths. Now she feels refreshed and alive, ready to face the afternoon.

After walking back to the office and up the stairs once more, Janice settles back down at her desk with her bottle filled with fresh water. For two minutes she closes her eyes and takes some deep breaths allowing her body to settle back into its natural rhythm. Then she opens her eyes and dives back into the projects on her desk.

About 2 p.m., Janice stops working to stand up and stretch a few times. Then she pulls out her bag of almonds along with a few baby carrots from the package she keeps in the office refrigerator. She munches nuts and veggies while sipping fresh water as she finishes up a few e-mails.

Later, about 3:30 p.m., Janice leaves her desk, walks downstairs to personally deliver a memo. She moves with determination, her body feels revived with nice, easy exercise. Back in the office she attends a brainstorming meeting for a new ad campaign. She sips water and treats herself to a piece of dark chocolate.

By 5 p.m., Janice has gotten in a good day's work and has also consumed the equivalent of 10 glasses of water, treated her body to fresh food and invigorating movement, and successfully kept stress at bay with plenty of short breaks and deep breathing. Satisfied with a job well done, she walks to her car and drives home, where her children have spent the afternoon playing outside with their neighbor and her three children.

After settling in at home, Janice quickly slices up some oranges for everyone, which they eat while they catch up on the events of the day. Then as the kids settle into their homework at the kitchen counter, Janice pulls together an easy dinner of broiled chicken, steamed asparagus, and sparkling water with a slice of lime. They finish with a dish of vanilla ice cream drizzled with honey and sliced strawberries.

Once dessert is done and the kids have finished clearing dishes, they all head outside to walk Buster around the block. Then, back in the house, they settle in front of the TV to watch their favorite sitcom.

At 9 p.m. it's off to bed for the kids and an hour in front of the computer for Janice, she's writing a couple personal e-mails while she pops a few frozen grapes from the freezer. She enjoys them with two more glasses of water before settling into bed with a novel she's been looking forward to reading.

At 10:30 p.m. her alarm goes off, reminding her it's time to put her book down and go to bed, otherwise she'd probably keep reading for hours, and pay for it in the morning. Despite being a single mom on a full schedule, Janice feels healthy, in control, and much more satisfied with her life.

Now *You* Are in Control

Give yourself a pat on the back, too. In the few hours it took to read this book, you've done more to ensure your health and quality of life than most people will do in a year. Now that you know how easy it is to work the *Simple Health Values* into your life without making painful sacrifices, it's up to you to simply respond with healthy actions.

With these five simple solutions, you're back in control of your own healthcare and healthy lifestyle. You now have the power to decide how healthy you'll feel, how often you'll get sick, how many times you'll need to see a doctor and even how good you'll look.

Relax, you don't need to jump into all five *Health Values* at once. Just try one to begin. Drink more water or eat more fresh foods. Try it, see how easy it is to do, and you'll begin to see the benefits. Then work another *Health Value* into your life. Before you know it, you'll be doing all five and you'll feel better than ever before.

Remember, *any* amount of forward momentum in simple health decisions is a success. And success is my hope for you.

Tools to Enhance Your
Simple Health Value Experience

General Information Websites

- Simple Health Value (www.simplehealthvalue.com)
- Alliance for Natural Health (www.alliance-natural-health.org)
- Worldwide Health Center (www.worldwidehealthcenter.net)
- Citizens for Health (www.citizens.org)
- Alternative Health News Online (www.altmedicine.com)
- Internet Health Library (www.internethealthlibrary.com)
- Holistic Health Network (www.holisticnetwork.org)
- About.com (healing.about.com)
- HerbalGram (www.herbalgram.org)
- Preferred Consumer (www.preferredconsumer.com/healthy_living)
- Campaign for Better Health (www.betterhealthcampaign.org)
- Council for Responsible Nutrition (www.crnusa.org)
- Find a Health Store (www.findahealthstore.com)
- WorldHealth.net (www.worldhealth.net)
- SupplementInfo.org (www.supplementinfo.org)
- Naturopathy Online (www.naturopathyonline.com)
- Whole Health MD (www.wholehealthmd.com)
- Healthwise (www.healthwise.org)
- Five to Ten a Day (www.5to10aday.com)
- America's Family of Pediatricians (www.askdrsears.com)
- Age Wave (www.agewave.com)

Magazines

- Alternative Medicine (www.alternativemedicine.com)
- Health (www.health.com)
- Cooking Light (www.cookinglight.com)
- Prevention (www.prevention.com)
- Better Nutrition (www.betternutrition.com)
- Real Simple (www.realsimple.com)
- Vegetarian Times (www.vegetariantimes.com)
- Eating Well (www.eatingwell.com)
- Vitality (www.vitality.com)
- Delicious Living (www.deliciouslivingmag.com)
- Body and Soul (www.bodyandsoulmag.com)

Books

- *Eat to Live, the Revolutionary Formula for Fast and Sustained Weight Loss*, by Joel Fuhrman, M.D.
- *NO More Heart Disease*, by Louis J. Ignarro, Ph.D.
- *Fresh Choices: More than 100 Easy Recipes for Pure Food When You Can't Buy 100% Organic*, by Rochelle Davis, David Joachim
- *Eat, Drink, and Be Healthy: The Harvard Medical School Guide to Healthy Eating*, by Walter Willett, M.D.
- *Living Foods for Optimum Health: Staying Healthy in an Unhealthy World*, by Theresa Foy Digeronimo, Brian R. Clement
- *Dr. Jensen's Nutrition Handbook: A Daily Regimen for Healthy Living*, by Bernard Jensen, Ph.D.
- *100 Simple Secrets of Healthy People: What Scientists Have Learned and How You Can Use it*, by David Niven
- *Cooking the Whole Foods Way*, by Christina Pirello

- *The Whole Food Bible: How to Select and Prepare Safe, Healthful Foods*, by Christopher Kilham
- *Healthy Habits: 20 Simple Ways to Improve Your Health*, by David J. Frahm and Anne Frahm
- *Your Body's Many Cries for Water*, by F. Batmanghelidj
- *Fast Food Nation: The Dark Side of the All-American Meal*, by Eric Schlosser
- *Nontoxic, Natural, & Earthwise*, by Debra Lynn Dadd
- *Herbal Prescriptions for Better Health*, by Donald J. Brown, N.D.
- *Encyclopedia of Natural Medicine*, by Michael T. Murray, N.D. and Joseph Pizzorno, N.D.
- *Nutritional Influences of Illness*, by Melvyn R. Werbach, M.D.
- *Encyclopedia of Nutritional Supplements*, by Michael T. Murray, N.D.
- *The Family Nutrition Book*, by William Sears, M.D. and Martha Sears, R.N.
- *Perfect Health*, by Deepak Chopra
- *Divided Legacy: The Conflict between Homeopathy and The American Medical Association*, by Harris L. Coulter
- *Reclaiming Our Health*, by John Robbins
- *Diet for a New America*, by John Robbins
- *Vibrational Medicine*, by Richard Gerber, M.D.
- *Age Wave: How the Most Important Trend of Our Time Will Change Your Future*, by Ken Dychtwald, Ph.D. and Joe Flower
- *Lifetime Physical Fitness and Wellness*, by Werner Hoeger

Organizations

- American Holistic Health Association (www.ahha.org)
- Organic Consumers Association (www.organicconsumers.org)
- National Health Federation (www.thenhf.com)
- Center for Science in the Public Interest (www.cspinet.org)

Naturopathic Physicians

- American Association of Naturopathic Physicians (www.naturopathic.org)

Please share your stories with us.

We would love to hear how
Simple Health Value has positively
impacted your life.

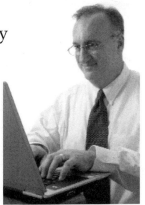

Submit your story or testimonial to:

www.simplehealthvalue.com/testimonials

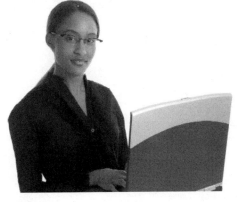

or mail to:

Health Value Publications
Attn: Simple Health Value
1810 W State #431
Boise, Idaho 83702

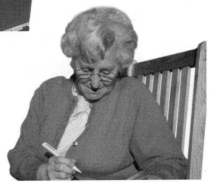

Bring bottom line health information to your company or organization.

Inquire about a live keynote presentation by Dr. Andrew Myers. He is able to share with executives, team leaders and employees the potential of simple actions to improve personal wellness and cut health care costs throughout the organization. He will provide your audience with new perspectives on productivity, individual and team performance with measurable benefits and powerful outcomes.

Meet the author in person and treat your group to the energy and impact of Dr. Myers' empowering presentations.

Book a keynote speech, corporate book signing, or live presentation. Contact Maryanna Young at maryanna@simplehealthvalue.com or 208 447 9036

Spread the word.

Simple Health Value books are available at quantity discounts for orders of 10 or more copies. Additional volume discounts apply for quantities of 100, 500 or 1000.

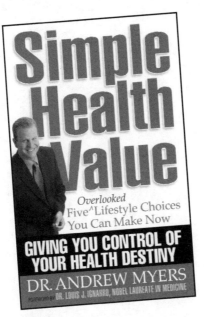

ISBN 978-0-9790229-0-6
Retail price $14.95 USA
$17.95 Canada

To find out about our discounts for orders of 10 or more copies for individuals, corporations, academic use, associations and organizations, please call us at **208 344 2733**.

To find out about our discount program for resellers, please contact our Special Sales department at **specialsales@simplehealthvalue.com**

Watch for upcoming *Simple Health Value*® books, workbooks, and daily tools for improving your health.

ABOUT THE AUTHOR

D r. Andrew Myers is one of those rare individuals who can see wellness solutions in aspects of medicine frequently overlooked by conventional care. A widely respected Naturopathic Medical Doctor, he is leading a long overdue effort to realign the foundations of health care and orient them where they belong—in our daily lifestyle choices.

The logical and practical recommendations in this book, reflect his belief that true wellness is achievable for everyone. Dr. Myers' passion is to help people understand how their lifestyle choices influence the function of their bodies and their direct impact on their lifelong health.

A graduate of Bastyr University, one of the world's leading academic centers for advancing knowledge in the natural health sciences, Dr. Myers strongly encourages changes in wellness habits for the prevention of devastating illnesses such as cardiovascular disease, cancer, diabetes and obesity. A down-to-earth, dynamic speaker, Dr. Myers connects with audiences with genuine passion and a straightforward message of empowerment.

Dr. Myers is currently the President and Chief Science Officer of Nutragenetics, a global product company founded by Nobel Laureate Dr. Lou Ignarro. He is also the Founder and CEO of Simple Health Value.